T010886?

The Nursing Mother's Herbal

The
NURSING MOTHER'S
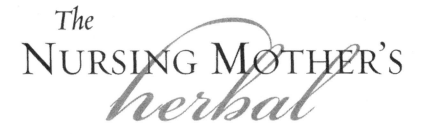

SHEILA HUMPHREY, BSc, RN, IBCLC

Fairview Press
Minneapolis

in cooperation with the
Center for Spirituality and Healing
University of Minnesota

The Nursing Mother's Herbal © 2003 Sheila Humphrey. All rights reserved. No part of this publication may be used or reproduced in any manner whatsoever without written permission, except in the case of brief quotations embodied in critical articles and reviews. For further information, please contact the publisher.

Published by Fairview Press (2450 Riverside Avenue, Minneapolis, Minnesota 55454), in cooperation with the Center for Spirituality and Healing, University of Minnesota. Fairview Press is a division of Fairview Health Services, a community-focused health system providing a complete range of services, from the prevention of illness and injury to care for the most complex medical conditions.

The Center for Spirituality and Healing

Established in 1995 at the University of Minnesota, the Center for Spirituality and Healing is a nationally recognized leader in mind-body medicine and brings together biomedical, complementary, cross-cultural, and spiritual aspects of patient care. For more information, go to www.csh.umn.edu.

ISBN-10: 1-57749-118-1
ISBN-13: 978-1-57749-118-7

Library of Congress Cataloging-in-Publication Data
Humphrey, Sheila, 1951–
  The nursing mother's herbal / Sheila Humphrey.
    p. cm. — (The human body library)
Includes bibliographical references and index.
  ISBN 1-57749-118-1—ISBN (invalid) 0-7660-2021-5
1. Breast feeding—Popular works. 2. Herbs—Therapeutic use—Popular works. 3. Materia medica, Vegetable—Toxicology—Popular works. I.
Title. II. Series.
RJ216.H855 2003
613.2'69—dc 21
                            2003009243

First Printing: November 2003
Printed in the United States of America

Cover: Laurie Ingram

For a free current catalog of Fairview Press titles, please call toll-free 1-800-544-8207. Or visit our website at www.fairviewpress.org.

Medical Disclaimer:
This publication is designed to provide accurate and authoritative information in regard to the subject matter covered. It is sold with the understanding that the publisher is not engaged in the provision or practice of medical, nursing, or professional healthcare advice or services in any jurisdiction. If medical advice or other professional assistance is required, the services of a qualified and competent professional should be sought. Neither Fairview Press nor the author is responsible or liable, directly or indirectly, for any form of damages whatsoever resulting from the use (or misuse) of information contained in or implied by these documents.

To my mother,
who gave me everything of importance;
to my older sister, Eleanor,
who taught a teenager that breastfeeding could be a joy;
and to my younger sister, Glenda,
who taught a beginner the finer points of counseling the nursing mother

Contents

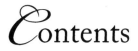

Acknowledgments

I would like to thank the plant people in my life, especially my parents and grandparents.

I would like to thank my professors of botany at the University of British Columbia—in particular, Robert DeWreede, for his patience, and Kay Beamish, whose first teaching on plant taxonomy was the observation that every new generation of living beings has been physically touched by their parents. We are the latest link in a continuous chain of physical connection stretching back to the very beginning of life on earth. I would also like to thank Dr. Neil Towers for his many gatherings of graduate students and visiting scholars. The food, music, and plant talk were always good, if, at times, a little wild.

Always, I am indebted to La Leche League, in more ways than I can begin to explain here. The organization has provided me information and support as a mother, Leader, and Leader assisting other Leaders.

I would like to thank the following women, who understand mother-to-mother helping so well: Sandee Luttkus, Betty Crase, Becky Hugh,

Linda Healow, Judy Minami, Carole Huotari, Carol Kolar, Kathy Parkes, Mary Kay Smith, Ghislaine Reid, Carrie Magill Vlastos, Sara Braveheart, Michele Lein, Kathleen Kendall-Tackett, Joan Balfour, Pat Gima, Beverley Morgan, Pam Galle, Aileen Emerling, Akane Kanamori, Hiroko Hongo, Nobuko Tsutsui, Cyndi Sherar, Deb Roberts, Kathleen Quarfordt, Jennifer Peddlesden, Diane West, Janet Gerla, Carmen Cabrerra, Elizabeth Hormann, Marty O'Donnell, Nancy Mohrbacher, and Julie Stock. My mother-models: Charlotte Burger (wherever you are), Kat Harrison, and Mary MacIntosh. A deep debt of gratitude goes to those with a special enthusiasm for the topic of herb use and breastfeeding who have so generously shared their expertise and perspectives: Mechell Turner, Kathryn Higgins, Diane Wiessinger, Jan Barger, Renate Rietveld, Gonneke van Veldhuizen, Donna Walls, Cheryl Renfree, Sharon Knorr, Pamela Morrison, Cindy Curtis, Ed Kasper, Françoise Railhet, Hilary Jacobson, Kathleen Huggins, Ulrike Schmidleithner, Jennifer Tow, Jay Gordon, Lisa Boisvert-McKenzie, Tami Karnes, Barbara Latterner, Pamela Berens, Nancy Hurst, Janet Talmadge, Kerry Luskey, Jamie Anderson, Kim Hedegaard, Eleanor Goldfarb, Jamie Otremba, Frank Nice, and Bob Longmore. Thanks to Jack Newman and Tom Hale, who had encouraging things to say at critical times, but even more for their generous gifts of information.

I am especially grateful for the "herb guys"—James Duke, Mark Blumenthal, and Andrew Weil—lovely, decent fellows, with a gift of writing in plain English. Jim must be especially acknowledged for his generous sharing of information over the years. Thanks also to Christopher Hafner-Eaton and the herb experts who gave me helpful feedback: Martha Libster, Roy Upton, Christopher Hobbs, Matthew Alfs, Tierona Low Dog, Aviva Romm, Hyla Cass, Sunny Mavor, Al Leung, and Ken Jones. Special thanks to Kat Harrison, who challenged me to stop complaining about the lack of information on herbs and lactation and get the book written.

I would like to thank Lane Stiles, my patient and encouraging publisher at Fairview Press, for his unflagging support. Many thanks for the extensive editing rendered by Elizabeth Verdick and Stephanie Billecke, who turned my tortured prose into something readable.

I would like to thank Mary Jo Kreitzer, Greg Plotnikoff, and the faculty of the Center for Spirituality and Healing at the University of Minnesota Academic Health Center for many opportunities to learn and for the Center's assistance in making this book a reality.

I would like to acknowledge how important my family has been in writing this book. The fact that my husband, Dennis McKenna, is a *PhD* botanist specializing in the study of medicinal plant pharmacology and ethnobotany has allowed me access to a vast store of botanical knowledge. He has been more than generous in sharing his expertise and research. Of equal importance are the irreplaceable contributions of my daughter, Caitlin. She was my best teacher about all things having to do with breastfeeding. Caitlin can be credited as well with providing a first-rate education on the exquisite interplay between temperament, breastfeeding, and parenting.

❦ ❦ ❦

This book is written in an easy-to-read format that does not include references in the text. For my sources, I have relied on the best current knowledge of lactation, pharmacology, botany, plant chemistry, toxicology, and herbalism, as well as the clinical experiences of both conventional and CAM practitioners. I refer readers to the standard reference texts listed in appendix A, from which most of the information was drawn. I have also relied on what mothers say about their experiences with herbs, even though most of this anecdotal evidence awaits scientific study. Science continues to affirm what mothers and their helpers have long known to be true about how breastfeeding works. A similar observation could be made of plant medicine: science continues to affirm the traditions of herbalism. I have strived to be an accurate messenger of existing knowledge and its applications, while being acutely aware of how much remains to be discovered.

Not everything that counts can be counted, and not everything that can be counted counts.

—Albert Einstein

Introduction

My parents were definitely plant people. As farmers in the interior dryland of British Columbia in western Canada, they knew a lot about the local plants and how to use them. They noticed plants and taught me to notice them, too. Their knowledge of plants was crucial to their survival. Our vegetable garden was not simply for fun—it was an integral part of our family economy, as were the alfalfa fields and the natural hay meadows from which we harvested hay to feed our sheep and cattle.

I absorbed plant lore by watching and helping my parents. I watched my dad irrigate the alfalfa, weed the garden, and pick the beans. He always had a big dried puffball mushroom in the barn because nothing stopped a cut from bleeding as quickly as the mushroom's dusty spores. I went with my mother to harvest wild mushrooms that grew in a special place at a special time each year. In summer, she would harvest watercress from a spring behind the barn to make wonderful sandwiches. She sent my sister and me out with pails to pick Saskatoon berries in late summer, telling us not to come back until we had enough to can for winter pies. We ate almost as many as we picked. My dad always warned us not to eat the snowberries on nearby bushes; years later, I learned that the local Salish Indian nation also considered these berries to be poisonous. I learned how chokecherries got their name (because they pucker your mouth, even as their natural sweetness makes you want to eat more). My parents made delicious chokecherry wine from the heavily laden bushes that grew luxuriously along the creeks. My parents also made dandelion wine. My dad always said that a small glass of dandelion wine was potent enough to keep you from getting out of your chair—and I found out this was true. His mother's dandelion wine recipe is a precious part of my inheritance.

My maternal grandmother, Nana, was an uneducated woman whose medicine did not include anything prescribed by a doctor. Nana stored dark brown smelly stuff in her bedroom closet, part of the mystery of her plant knowledge. She kept a huge garden from which most of her food was grown, including mysterious gooseberries and other unusual plants. Long before I'd ever heard of "health food," Nana was juicing her own garden carrots to drink every day. She was the only person I knew who ate avocados, a food I'd never seen nor heard of until she brought one to the dinner table and proceeded to eat it in front of us with obvious relish. To her, an avocado was a special treat; but to my rural Canadian teenage mind, eating the green, oily flesh was too weird to imagine at the time. (To this day, every time I eat an avocado I think of her.) Nana's botanical adventures opened a door beyond my rural home to a wider world of plants, and she taught me by example what it means to have a relationship with plants. Whenever I wonder where I got my interest in botany, these memories and a thousand others from my childhood flood my mind.

I think that everyone is potentially a plant person. Children have a natural curiosity about plant life, and they remember well the plant lore they've been taught. Perhaps someone once showed you how to snap a snapdragon, or shared the story of the bleeding heart, or told you how to open a pea pod to eat the peas. For some of us, learning about plant lore and the healing properties of plants opens up a place in our hearts where the plant lives forever after. This was true for me.

After my first year of university sciences, I became smitten with botany. I earned a bachelor of science degree in botany and studied the natural history of every kind of plant—from mosses to algae to ferns—as well as their ecology, evolution, and economic importance. My work in graduate school was focused on plant ecology; while there, I met my future husband, who was studying an Amazonian medicinal brew of plants known as *ayuahuasca*. He and other botanists studying medicinal plants refamiliarized me with the idea of plants as a potential healing force. I grew even more interested in the medicinal uses of plants after hearing a lecture by Dr. Andrew Weil in the 1970s. Even then a masterful lecturer, he impressed upon me the idea that medicinal plants were not only fascinating in themselves but were an untapped reservoir for scientific and medical research. In the twenty-five years since, much research has been done throughout the world on the medicinal uses of plants. Yet, human knowledge about the use of plants in healing is far from complete; in the case of most traditional healing plants, medical research has barely begun.

I eventually decided to go into nursing as a profession. After my training, I worked in hospitals in Canada, California, and Washington, D.C. My husband, meanwhile, began working in the pharmaceutical and herb industry as an ethnobotanist and plant pharmacologist. When our daughter was born, I stayed home to care for her and soon became involved in the breastfeeding support organization known as La Leche League. I have been a Leader, or lay counselor, with this organization for thirteen years and subsequently certified as an International Board Certified Lactation Consultant (IBCLC) in 1996.

Over the years, I have helped other Leaders provide information to mothers who want to know about the use of medicines while breastfeeding. While studying drugs and breastfeeding, I became curious about medicinal plants and how they might affect nursing mothers and their babies. My husband's growing library of medicinal plant information soon drew my curiosity, but I found very little information and almost no research about breastfeeding in this literature. I was surprised at the lack of reliable information, and I decided to devote more time to the study of this neglected, but important, topic.

❧ ❧ ❧

Many people around the world are taking a greater interest in nutrition and how it connects to the prevention of illness. Studies have repeatedly shown that eating plenty of fruits and vegetables can protect our health in so many ways. We generally understand that these foods—these *plants*—contain the vitamins, minerals, and fiber we need to maintain our health, but we're still learning about how they protect us from certain illnesses. Today, we take for granted that eating foods containing vitamin C is vital for our health, and we may forget that, for many centuries, people died from scurvy, an illness caused by insufficient vitamin C. Although it had been widely known for at least two hundred years that eating foods such as citrus fruits prevented scurvy, the role that vitamin C played wasn't identified until much later.

What other diseases may eventually be attributed to nutritional deficiencies? Time alone will tell. We are still very much in the process of investigating the healing properties of plant foods and herbs. We have much to learn about how to use them in our daily lives and in modern medicine.

It's true that an ounce of prevention is worth a pound of cure. Investing a bit of time and effort in healthy life choices—for example, a sensible diet, regular exercise, and relaxation—can provide actual health benefits, both short- and long-term. And nowhere is this more evident than in feeding breast milk to babies. Sometimes called "Nature's Health Plan," breastfeeding is natural and normal for both mother and child, and the benefits for both cannot be overstated. Unfortunately, not everyone is as informed about these benefits as they should be.

This book was written to provide much needed information about the safe use of herbs when breastfeeding: safe use for the baby, but also for the mother and for breastfeeding itself. It seeks to educate about the benefits as well as the potential risks from using herbs while breastfeeding. Intended primarily for nursing mothers and their helpers as a basic introduction to healing plants and their use as food and medicine, *The*

Nursing Mother's Herbal also aims to help nursing mothers prevent or find solutions for health problems that they or their babies may experience during breastfeeding.

Please keep in mind that this book is not a substitute for medical attention. Should you experience any severe, unusual, or persistent symptoms, consult your healthcare provider immediately. The more serious and complex your health condition, the more important it is that you seek the advice of a medical doctor. If possible, consult a doctor who is knowledgeable about and supportive of nursing. A physician who is also open to and informed about alternative or complementary medicine can also be a valuable asset as you consider treatment options. Be sure to let your doctor know about any treatments or medicinal agents you are using, whether or not the physician is providing these treatments.

🌿 🌿 🌿

As you feed your baby, you provide health benefits for both your baby and yourself. Breastfeeding is a challenge that, when met successfully, will help you feel strong and proud. You will define for yourself what successful breastfeeding means for you and your child, but it's worth celebrating anytime you feed breast milk to your baby. While nursing, you will discover that you yourself are a force for good health. Just watch how big, beautiful, and healthy your baby becomes with your milk. Any amount of breastfeeding brings health.

As with any endeavor, having the encouragement of loved ones will help. Talk to your partner and family members about nursing and how they may best support you during this time. Find other nursing mothers who can share their information and tips with you. This will help you feel more supported and nourished as you nourish your baby.

🌿 🌿 🌿

Many of you may have already heard or read about the health benefits of breastfeeding, or know them firsthand. But perhaps you haven't yet found a reliable source of information about what is safe to ingest while breastfeeding. Vitamins? Herbs? Medications? Prescription drugs? Which substances may be harmful—and which ones can be helpful or healing? Which foods and herbs can help promote a better breastfeeding experience? This book is a guide to all of these questions and more.

Perhaps you have a health issue that needs treatment and you've been advised to wean your baby. If this is the case, you may doubt whether weaning is truly the best course of action (and rightly so, when breastfeeding provides proven health benefits for you and your baby). As a nursing mother, you have the right to ask important questions: Is weaning really best? Why or why not? What are the risks of weaning? What are the benefits of continuing to breastfeed? What other treatment choices do I have? Where is the information that supports my choices and options?

Many healthcare providers and other experts warn nursing mothers that the substances they ingest will be "risky" for the baby. Yet, in reality, weaning may actually be the riskier choice. Most prescription drugs and over-the-counter (OTC) medications are considered compatible with breastfeeding, a fact recently noted in *Pediatrics,* a journal published by the American Academy of Pediatrics (AAP).[1] Research spanning the past twenty years has shown that a drug's dose in breast milk is so small that there will be little or no effect on the baby. There are exceptions, of course, and these have been well documented.

Likewise, many herbs and healing plants are generally safe for nursing mothers and their babies. But as a nursing mother, you need specific information about what to expect when taking an herb or any other natural substance. Will use of it help or hinder breastfeeding? How much of the herb should you take and when should you take it? What effect might it have on your baby or your milk supply? What are the known benefits or risks? Are there safer alternatives? *The Nursing Mother's Herbal* will help you answer these questions—and know what questions to ask.

$\mathcal{B}$reastfeeding

Just as cow's milk best serves a calf (and mouse's milk a baby mouse), a mother's breast milk best meets the nutritional needs of her infant. For hundreds of thousands of years, babies breastfed right from birth. There simply was no other way to feed infants before formulas derived from cow's milk were developed. Today's babies still have the needs that the first human infants had following birth: oxygen, their mothers, the breast, and breast milk.

As surely as he* takes a breath after his first exposure to air, a baby nurses in response to meeting the breast. He starts his amazing development using all of his new abilities. His first breath allows him to smell his mother; his first motions serve to move him up to her breast and, seeing the darker areola, to latch on. His very first taste of breast milk provides an immediate dose of infection-fighting antibodies. The small but vital amount of colostrum (first milk) he receives after birth

---

*Throughout the book, I will refer to the breastfeeding baby as "he" and to the nursing mother as "she." I will do this to make the text simpler and more straightforward.

stabilizes his blood sugar; his mother's body warms him. In these ways, he survives the first hours after birth, a time when his ability to maintain his blood sugar and body warmth are limited.

The warming contact with his mother, provided by early feedings at the breast, help ensure a successful transition to life outside the womb. Rhythmic sucking comforts him after his placid life in utero. And the food! Breast milk is the sole nutritional source needed for many months to come. It is sweet, it is warm, and it tastes different every day.

Of course, there is more to life than food and warmth. The equally vital needs for contact, love, and communication are met through nursing at the breast. A mother's desire to touch and communicate with her baby, as well as to feed him, are also met through nursing. Breastfeeding can be a pleasurable, fulfilling experience that helps a mother and her baby grow closer and begin to establish a loving, lifelong bond.

The Health Benefits of Breastfeeding

Simply put, lactation is a natural part of the reproductive process; breastfeeding is meant to follow pregnancy and birth. Both the mother's and the baby's bodies are biologically prepared for nursing. But just how important is breastfeeding? And just what is actually at stake? Consider the proven health benefits.

For Mothers

- Placing an infant to the breast right away encourages the uterus to contract after childbirth, helping to prevent postpartum hemorrhage. Nursing keeps the uterus well contracted, which helps a mother to more quickly regain her pre-pregnant shape.

- Mothers who nurse can expect a delay in the return of ovulation and menstrual periods after childbirth. The Lactation Amenorrhea Method (LAM), based on exclusive breastfeeding, is a well-researched and effective birth control method promoted by the World Health Organization (WHO) and used successfully around the world. Mothers who breastfeed exclusively can expect a delay in ovulation of at least six months.

• Breastfeeding uses calories and alters metabolism in other ways, so nursing mothers return to their pre-pregnant weight more quickly.

• Mothers who breastfeed tend to have stronger bones. While their bone density may be temporarily lowered during nursing, after weaning their bone density increases and their bones may even become stronger than they were before the mothers became pregnant.

• Breastfeeding lowers the risk of developing breast and ovarian cancers, a fact recently recognized by the American Academy of Pediatrics. A number of studies have shown a reduction in the occurrence of these cancers in women who have breastfed; the longer they nursed, the less their risk of these diseases.

• Breastfeeding women develop greater self-esteem and assertiveness, become more outgoing, and become more active in the development and management of their own lives.[2]

For Infants

• Breastfeeding prevents or lessens the severity of eczema, asthma, severe allergies including food allergies, and other hypersensitivity conditions. There is also a lowered risk of developing celiac disease, appendicitis, or severe liver disease.

• Breastfeeding is associated with a lower lifetime risk of autoimmune diseases such as insulin-dependent diabetes, Crohn's disease, and rheumatoid arthritis.

• Diarrhea, ear infections, respiratory illnesses such as RSV (respiratory syncytial virus), pneumonia, meningitis, botulism, and urinary tract infections are prevented or lessened in severity among babies who breastfeed.

- Breastfed babies are less likely to be hospitalized as a result of illness.

- Breastfed babies hardly ever experience constipation or anemia.

- The breastfed baby, with his more competent immune system, has a fuller response to vaccines for polio, tetanus, whooping cough, and diphtheria and is able to make more antibodies compared to babies who are fed formula.

- Premature infants who are fed breast milk are much less likely to develop necrotizing enterocolitis, a potentially deadly bowel complication.

- Breastfed babies are less likely to succumb to Sudden Infant Death Syndrome (SIDS).

- Breastfeeding helps the jaw, teeth, and facial muscles of the baby to develop more normally. (Babies must use their jaw, tongue, and facial muscles differently to drink from a bottle.) Proper jaw development is associated with fewer speech problems and less of a need for orthodontic treatment later in life.

- Breastfeeding may help prevent the onset of adult sleep apnea. Some researchers associate adult sleep apnea with an underdeveloped jaw and the resultant narrowed airway passages seen in bottle-fed populations.

- Breastfeeding leads to normal weight gain in infants and helps guard against obesity later in life. A recent study clearly showed that babies who were breastfed exclusively for approximately six months and who continued to breastfeed into their second year had the lowest incidence of obesity as teenagers.

- Breastfeeding lowers the likelihood of developing certain childhood cancers.

- Being fed breast milk decreases a female baby's risk of developing breast cancer as an adult.

- Breastfed babies achieve a significantly higher degree of visual and intellectual development than formula-fed babies. Lower visual and cognitive ability, and lowered IQ have repeatedly been measured in infants, children, and adults who were fed formula.

For all of these reasons and more, breastfeeding provides a lifetime of benefits for you and your child. In the words of La Leche League, it is "the best start in life for a baby. Unlike so much that is considered 'best' and is often beyond even one's wildest dreams, in this instance the best is yours to give." [3]

The Health Risks of Baby Formulas

In the United States today, whenever breast milk isn't available, formula is always at hand, and its use is commonly considered "almost as good as" breast milk—despite twenty years of research showing otherwise. Ads in parenting magazines and on television promote baby formula as "the next best thing to breast milk," convincing many parents that formula feeding is a healthy alternative. Yet, it is actually a poor *fourth* choice, according to Dr. Jack Newman, a Canadian pediatrician and an internationally recognized expert on breastfeeding and lactation. Here is how he ranks baby-feeding options:

1. Nursing at the breast is best.

2. Feeding with a mother's expressed breast milk is next best.

3. Feeding with donated expressed breast milk is next after that.

4. Baby formula is a last resort (due to loss of human milk benefits and the inherent risk of formulas).[4]

The World Health Organization also disagrees that formula feeding is the next best thing to breastfeeding. The World Health Organization and UNICEF put forth this statement: "Give newborn infants no food or drink other than breast milk, unless medically indicated.... The administration by bottle or teat of water, herbal teas, glucose solutions, or worse still, milk-based formulas not only is unnecessary on nutritional grounds but reduces the infant's sucking capacity and therefore the mother's lactation stimulus. Furthermore, such practices increase the risk of introducing infection and, in the case of milk-based formulas, of sensitizing an infant to cow's milk protein."[5] The World Health Organization specifically recommends breastfeeding for two years and beyond.

Research has shown that donated milk has far fewer risks than baby formula and is a very cost-effective form of preventive medicine. Expressed breast milk has anti-infective properties that greatly slow the rate of bacterial growth; the expressed milk also contains the best nutritional substances and requires little energy or raw materials in its manufacture. Expressed breast milk can easily be made sterile without the loss of most of its many unique benefits. (It is the only donated human substance that can be made sterile before use.) While donated milk is currently limited to feeding premature babies or those with other pressing nutritional needs—mainly because of a lack of funding for milk banks and a curious reluctance of doctors—many babies the world over could benefit from its use. In some European countries, most notably Sweden, all hospitalized babies are given human milk whether or not their mothers are breastfeeding; milk banking with donated milk ensures optimal nutrition for these babies in great need of the best.

The superiority of breast milk is in the milk itself, as well as in the act of feeding at the breast. Mothers and babies who exclusively breast-feed in the early months and continue breastfeeding for at least a year gain more health benefits and protection from illness and disease. In other words, the longer they breastfeed the more benefits they receive. Those who breastfeed for a shorter period of time gain smaller, but still real and measurable, benefits. On the other hand, babies who don't nurse receive none of the protections of breast milk. Their mothers don't reap the health rewards that nursing can provide, either.

Historically, a number of physicians have advocated breast milk over the formulas of their time. In a wonderful book called *Green Pharmacy: A History of Herbal Medicine*, author Barbara Griggs notes that a historic figure in herbal medicine, Samuel Coffin, not only recommended herbs, whole foods, and exercise, but also concluded that it was "absolute folly

What Do Pediatricians Now Recommend?

In 2002, the American Academy of Pediatrics made the following recommendations (heartily endorsed by breastfeeding experts) about the proper nutrition of infants and children:

1. Mothers should begin breastfeeding as soon as possible after birth, usually within the first hour.
2. Exclusive breastfeeding is best (no supplementing with formula or water) for about the first six months of life.
3. Breastfeeding for at least twelve months provides optimal health benefits.
4. After twelve months, breastfeeding may continue for as long as desired by the mother and her child.[6]

for infants to be fed anything other than breast milk."[7] What was clear to Dr. Coffin in the 1850s seems today to be less important in modern societies that have access to clean drinking water and the sterile preparation of baby formula. Although the use of modern baby formulas peaked in the 1970s, many parents and healthcare professionals still believe that feeding babies with bottles of formula is a healthy alternative.

Baby formulas are highly processed, factory-made products. The stakes are high when it comes to these formulas because infants may consume nothing but one brand for many months. What if a batch has been mixed incorrectly, with too much or too little of important ingredients? What about the risk of bacterial contamination when filling baby bottles? What if a powdered formula is combined at home with water that isn't safe to drink? Unfortunately, dangers such as these occur all too frequently. The truth is, even today, baby formula is a poor alternative to pure and time-tested mother's milk.

Successful Breastfeeding

HOW TO BUILD A SUPPORT NETWORK

Throughout your pregnancy, you have many things on your mind: taking good care of yourself, eating healthy for the baby, preparing your home for his arrival. Then, of course, there's labor and childbirth to consider! When you're focused on bringing your child into the world, it may be difficult to think past this point. However, it's important to prepare yourself for breastfeeding so you're ready once the moment arrives. If you're a first-time mother, take some time to learn about breastfeeding before you have your baby. Even if you're already a mom and have nursed previously, you may want to brush up on some breastfeeding basics.

This isn't a how-to chapter with breastfeeding techniques—there are already many wonderful books available that can help you learn how to nurse your baby. (You'll find a list of them in appendix A.) Instead, this chapter is designed to help you build a network of supporters who can give you the guidance and information you may need as a nursing mother. You'll learn how to get breastfeeding off to a good start and keep things on track—before your baby even arrives.

Read about Breastfeeding

If you're looking for a how-to book on nursing, I highly recommend *The Womanly Art of Breastfeeding*—the original (and still the best) breastfeeding manual. This fully revised and updated manual, published by La Leche League International, is the most informative book of its kind. There are many other good books on breastfeeding, but if you're not sure where to begin, consider reading some of those listed in appendix A. Ask other nursing mothers about books they recommend as well.

As you read about breastfeeding, you may come across magazine articles or web sites on the topic. Always consider whether the source is reputable. Does the article or web site appear to be current, accurate, and supportive of breastfeeding? Where does the information come from—a breastfeeding expert? a medical doctor? a company that produces baby formula? To ensure that you get the best guidance, look for web sites, magazines, or books that have been recommended by La Leche League Leaders, experienced nursing mothers, or other reputable sources.

Seek Out Nursing Mothers

A picture is worth a thousand words. Watching a mother nursing her baby can teach you more than you may think. Most nursing mothers will be glad to talk to you about their experiences and tell you what they've learned. Listening to their stories can light the road ahead.

Ask your own mother, aunts, or grandmothers about their experiences. They may have already told you their birth stories; now listen for their tales of breastfeeding. The wisdom of their experience can guide you. Or talk to friends and coworkers about their breastfeeding stories. Remember the stories of those who were happy to breastfeed and who did so with success.

Reading, watching, talking, listening—all of these things can help you prepare to breastfeed your baby. Learn from mothers who understand the joys and challenges of nursing a baby. They will be interested in helping you have a successful breastfeeding experience.

Using Herbs and Other Supplements during Pregnancy

During pregnancy, there are a few things to keep in mind to help breastfeeding get off to a good start. If you're using herbs to prepare for birth, consider discontinuing those that may increase your milk supply a couple weeks before birth. Herbs such as nettle or alfalfa may contribute to an overabundant milk supply or increased engorgement after birth. (Chapter 7 discusses milk supply; chapter 8 has information on engorgement.) It is best to ask a lactation specialist for guidance in your particular situation.

According to some recent studies, a baby's allergies may start during pregnancy. Eating a varied diet during your pregnancy can reduce the risk of sensitizing your baby to certain foods. Consider regularly supplementing your diet with yogurt or kefir (a yogurt beverage), or using probiotic capsules during your pregnancy, especially if you need an antibiotic. The beneficial bacteria in these products prevent bacterial and yeast infections from developing. Such infections inflame the gastrointestinal tract, making the tissues "leaky" or more permeable. The inflammation allows more allergenic proteins to enter your bloodstream, where they can be passed on to your growing baby. Using probiotics after birth may be helpful in preventing allergies in your baby, too.

If you have a family history of allergy, eczema, or autoimmune disease or if you already have a child with any of these conditions, you might consider adding enzyme supplements to your diet. They can help your body more completely digest proteins so that fewer enter your bloodstream from the GI tract. For more information, talk to a lactation specialist or a healthcare provider who is knowledgeable about these supplements. You can also read chapter 6, which covers postpartum nutrition, as well as chapters 7 and 8, which discuss milk supply and

Organize Your Breastfeeding Helpers

Many mothers have found that organizing their support system ahead of time is a great way to prepare. Before your baby is born, identify your breastfeeding helpers. Family members and friends who have breastfed can be of assistance, but you'll need other supporters, too. Your obstetrician or midwife, your regular healthcare provider, and your child's pediatrician should all be your allies. Find out if they have experience with nursing mothers; ask them how to get breastfeeding off to a good start and what they know about assisting with breastfeeding problems. Take a look at chapter 5 for information on finding providers who are knowledgeable and supportive.

It can be very helpful to attend a breastfeeding support meeting in your community so you can meet the mothers and counselors. This will make it easier to call on their help if you should ever need it. Try to get to know some mothers who are currently breastfeeding, who have breastfed successfully, and who can encourage your efforts. In particular, talk to mothers who have breastfed their children for at least a year. (The American Academy of Pediatrics now recommends breastfeeding for one year—read more about this in chapter 1.) Mothers who have nursed this long gain lots of insight. What worked for them may work for you, too.

Women at breastfeeding support meetings can refer you to supportive, informed healthcare providers in your area and tell you which doctors, clinics, and hospitals (in their experience) have been helpful with breastfeeding. If you're interested in alternative practitioners, alternative healing practices, or sources of whole foods and supplements, talk to the women at the meeting to find out whom, or what, they recommend.

Find a Lactation Specialist

Many women begin breastfeeding with the best of intentions but stop after a few days, weeks, or months. They switch to baby formula because they have run into a breastfeeding problem that they aren't sure how to handle. There are experts who are ready and willing to help you with such problems. Knowing who the experts are ahead of time can be your lifeline should difficulties arise.

This book uses the general term "lactation specialist" to refer to anyone who has a broad knowledge of breastfeeding, a helpful attitude combined with counseling skills, and a keen interest in protecting, promoting, and supporting breastfeeding. A lactation specialist may be a doctor, a nurse, or other healthcare professional, or may be an experienced nursing mother who has volunteered her time to help other mothers with breastfeeding. How, then, can you identify a qualified specialist in breastfeeding? There are two internationally protected and accredited lactation specialist titles:

- International Board Certified Lactation Consultant (IBCLC)

- La Leche League Leader (LLLL), a volunteer counselor
  accredited through La Leche League International

Experts with these titles will be your most reputable sources of breastfeeding help. You can rely on their extensive knowledge and trust that they are fully supportive of a mother's efforts to breastfeed.

International Board Certified Lactation Consultants

The International Lactation Consultant Association (ILCA) is a global professional organization that determines the scope and standards of practice for an International Board Certified Lactation Consultant. IBCLCs often practice in hospitals; usually, they are also registered nurses. IBCLCs might be dietitians, doctors, psychologists, or members of any other helping profession, however. International Board Certified Lactation Consultants don't need another professional license or other certification to become IBCLCs. They are part of your healthcare team and are paid for their services. Consider their fee a worthy investment in your child's future.

Anyone can call herself a "lactation consultant." The title isn't protected and doesn't guarantee that the person using it knows anything about breastfeeding or how to effectively support a nursing mother.

Many registered nurses in hospitals are referred to as the "lactation nurse" or "lactation consultant," but may not have gone through the prescribed training or taken the examination to earn the title of IBCLC. The preferred lactation specialists have (1) accreditation by internationally known and respected entities, (2) a base of knowledge about breastfeeding, and (3) helpful attitudes and counseling skills.

This isn't to say that registered nurses can't help—many of them have breastfed their own children successfully and possess the knowledge to assist you with a breastfeeding problem. Just because your wise neighbor who has several breastfed children isn't an IBCLC doesn't mean she can't help, either. However, if you're experiencing a problem with breastfeeding, time is of the essence. You may need the help of an expert who knows just what to do in your situation and can help you get back on track quickly and effectively.

La Leche League Leaders

La Leche League International is a nonprofit organization dedicated to providing information and free breastfeeding counseling to all mothers who want to breastfeed their babies. The focus of the organization is mother-to-mother support.

La Leche League Leaders are accredited lay counselors who have extensive personal experience; they breastfed exclusively for around six months and continued breastfeeding for at least a year after the introduction of solid foods. Leaders know the basics of breastfeeding, and they are taught group-management and counseling skills. As Leaders, they help with breastfeeding problems but assume that breastfeeding will continue—this unspoken attitude that weaning is a distant goal has helped many a mother find a way to solve a breastfeeding problem instead of giving up.

To learn more about La Leche League, visit the web site: www.lalecheleague.org. There is a hotline you can call as well: 1-800-LALECHE (from 9 A.M. to 3 P.M., Monday through Friday). A whole lot of healing happens over the phone. Many nursing mothers have been able to overcome breastfeeding challenges on their own when given some information and support.

Other Lactation Titles

Private companies accredit titles such as Credited Lactation Educator (CLE) or Credited Lactation Counselor (CLC). The companies and titles are not associated with the International Lactation Consultant Association or connected with nonprofit organizations such as La Leche League. People who have the titles CLE or CLC may be able to help you, but they will not necessarily have the educational preparation of Leaders or IBCLCs.

A Few Breastfeeding Basics

Even if you are totally prepared to nurse your baby, you may feel overwhelmed and confused once you put your newborn to your breast. It may seem that there are so many things to remember, or that your situation is different from those you've read or heard about. Be assured that in almost all situations, breastfeeding can be made to work for you and your baby—even if there are special circumstances such as a health issue. (Read more about special circumstances later in this chapter.) If you're a first-time mother, it may take some time to get breastfeeding to go smoothly; but chances are, you and your baby will get the hang of it. A little information and support can turn things around, especially if you seek help early on.

There are a few simple things to keep in mind as you and your baby start learning about breastfeeding.

Early and Often

Babies learn to breastfeed at the breast (a simple enough idea). This means it's best to put your baby to your breast right away—a few moments after birth, if possible. La Leche League believes that mothers should nurse their babies early and often so that both mother and baby can get a running start on learning about latching onto the breast. Nursing early is also important because this allows the baby to take in colostrum, or first milk, which is filled with antibodies and other infection-fighting cells. The colostrum helps a baby to quickly pass meconium, the black sticky stool that is in his gastrointestinal tract at birth.

At the earliest stage of breastfeeding, your breasts will be softer; within a few days, large volumes of milk will automatically start to be produced, and some engorgement (or a lot) will start to make your breasts firmer, or even hard. If you get lots of practice with nursing when your breasts are still producing colostrum, you may have an easier time once your milk comes in. Nursing frequently in the early days not only helps prevent painful engorgement but also goes a long way toward establishing a good milk supply.

Focus on Latching

Latching refers to how a baby takes the nipple and areola into his mouth. A good latch will mean a more successful breastfeeding experience. In the beginning, many babies have a less-than-perfect latch. The early days of nursing are learning days for both mother and baby.

Positioning your baby for breastfeeding may seem awkward at first, even if you've observed other nursing mothers. It takes a certain amount of care, attention, and patience. One general principle holds true for all positions and latching methods: however they latch, babies need to get a good mouthful of the breast to be able to extract milk well.

Tenderness and some pain with initial latching are very common; these symptoms tend to ease up once the milk starts flowing. But soreness that persists between feedings indicates that something is hurting the nipple. Almost always, fixing the latch will fix the soreness.

If the nipples crack or bleed—which can happen very quickly—it may be because the baby isn't latching and nursing correctly. If the breasts become painfully engorged and nursing does not bring relief, this may also be because the baby is not latching correctly and removing enough milk. Review your breastfeeding information for positioning and latching to see if something obvious can be fixed. If things don't improve within a few days of adjusting your baby's latch, get some help right away. (See chapter 8 for more information about sore nipples and engorgement.)

There are many illustrated books about breastfeeding that discuss positioning and latching in detail. Videos are also available, so contact a lactation specialist or check out La Leche League's group library. It's always helpful to watch other women breastfeeding their children, too. Many mothers find it helpful to keep their favorite breastfeeding manual close at hand, so they can refer to it often in the early days and weeks of nursing.

Self-attachment

Some hospitals recommend that the baby go skin-to-skin on the mother's belly immediately after birth so that he has the opportunity to nurse before receiving other routine care. This process is called "self-attachment." Assuming there are no medical difficulties for either the mother or the baby, the baby is placed on the mother's belly immediately after birth and covered with a light blanket. Usually, the baby will make kicking motions and push himself up to his mother's breast. He will bob his head and eventually find the nipple and begin to nurse. The process can take up to an hour, so patience and trust are needed. Self-attachment, as described here, is not encouraged at every hospital. However, if you are planning to give birth at home with a midwife, you may want to talk about this option with her.

If you're not satisfied with how breastfeeding is going and you're not sure what to do, look to your support network. It may take about a month to six weeks before you get to a point where breastfeeding comes easily at every feeding, but there will be a day when you won't need three pillows and several tries just to get the baby latched. For some mothers this day comes sooner—every baby is different.

What Goes In Must Come Out

Babies nurse, on average, about eight to twelve times per day. However, newborns and some older babies may want to nurse more often than this, and a few thrive while nursing only every three or four hours. Every mother and baby are unique. If only you could see the milk going in. This would ease any worries about whether your baby is feeding enough. For many mothers, this is the number one concern about breastfeeding, and the number one reason for quitting. Rest assured—the amount of milk that goes in your baby will determine how much comes out the other end, so you have a way to monitor how much he consumes. A simple review of the contents of your baby's diapers will tell you if he is getting enough to eat.

In the first three to four days after your baby is born, the rule of thumb is that he should have one wet diaper for each day after birth. This shows that he is getting the all-important colostrum.

Before your milk comes in, your baby will have few wet or soiled diapers; but once the large volumes of milk start flowing, you should notice a dramatic change in your baby's output. The number of wet diapers should increase, and the meconium should rapidly change from black to golden; its consistency will be somewhat liquid.

Within just a couple days of increased milk production, the amount of dirty diapers will increase. During those first few days, your baby's stools will be greenish black or tarry looking, but by about the third day, they should start to become much lighter or greenish in color. Within one to two days of your milk coming in, your baby should have at least three to four bowel movements every day. He should also produce lots of wet diapers—a sign that he is well hydrated. Look for at least six to eight really wet cloth diapers, or five to six really wet disposable diapers.

Your baby may lose up to 10 percent of his birth weight in the first three to four days of life. But after your milk comes in, you can expect him to gain about four to eight ounces per week, or at least a pound a month. After six weeks of age, many babies start to have fewer stools but continue to gain weight well. A few signs of a healthy baby: he will appear active and alert, his skin will be firm and have a good color, and he will outgrow his newborn clothes. If your baby doesn't seem to be gaining weight, it's important to talk to his doctor and get breastfeeding help from someone who is skilled in this area. Don't delay.

If your baby's doctor suggests weaning or supplementing with formula, ask how else your breastfeeding problem can be solved. Seek expert help as soon as possible if your baby's doctor continues to encourage weaning. Sometimes, it is necessary to use baby formula if your child is hungry, but formula is rarely needed for long. Remember that you can express your milk to feed your baby, which is better than feeding your baby formula. Expressing milk also stimulates your breasts to make more milk. Simply adding formula will decrease your baby's interest in feeding and lower your supply. Do all you can to continue with breastfeeding. Even if things get off to a rough start, there are many ways to get back on track, and people willing to help you do it.

Promoting a Good Supply

Your breasts have the ability to make lots of milk (enough for twins, if needed), but this initial supply can diminish within a couple of weeks. This is why it's important to establish a good milk supply early on.

Breastfeeding works on supply and demand. As your baby removes milk from your breasts, they are stimulated to make more for the next feeding. On days when your baby is especially hungry, he will nurse more often and you will automatically make more milk in response. A good supply is established based on the baby's feeding cues and regular emptying of the breasts. If milk isn't removed on a regular basis, the milk supply goes down.

You can help ensure an adequate milk supply by nursing early and often, fixing a poor latch as soon as possible, and checking that your baby has frequent bowel movements and wet diapers. Remember, milk must come out of the breast for more milk to be made. Frequent removal of milk from the breast—either by nursing, using a breast pump, or expressing by hand—will help you build and keep a good supply. The goal is to breastfeed or express milk about eight to twelve times in a twenty-four-hour period (every two to three hours, with at least one session during the night). You may start out feeling that you are nursing all the time, but things do settle down—as much as this is possible with a new baby. For more about milk supply, see chapter 7.

Special Circumstances

If your circumstances are more complicated, I would encourage you to seek out someone who is knowledgeable about breastfeeding to discuss the situation. Find out how breastfeeding may be different for you and your baby. In most cases, breastfeeding *is* still possible.

Breastfeeding Multiples

While it may seem difficult, many mothers have exclusively breastfed their twins with success. Many mothers have even been able to breast-feed triplets (or more) at the breast, at least partially. If you're a mother of multiples, information and support are very important; so is finding expert assistance, especially in the early stages of breastfeeding. Mothers of multiples know that breastfeeding success takes many forms and may be achieved in a number of ways.

These days, you can find breastfeeding books written just for mothers of multiples. But these books are no substitute for talking with someone who has firsthand experience. You can learn so much from other mothers who have found ways to breastfeed multiples—their stories may inspire you, too. La Leche League may be able to put you in touch with a Leader or another mother who has had this special experience. Plan to find a circle of support when you're pregnant, as these helpers will be invaluable when your babies arrive. See appendices A and B for books and organizations that can help.

Breastfeeding the Baby with Health Problems

La Leche League has many resources to help mothers breastfeed or provide breast milk for special babies. In fact, the organization may be able to help you locate Leaders who have worked with mothers in similar situations, or who have breastfed children with the same health issue.

When a baby is born premature or has a problem, the medical team concentrates on his immediate health needs. Sometimes, the focus on establishing and maintaining a good milk supply is lost or forgotten. But for babies who are born early or are at risk because of health problems, breastfeeding becomes even more important. You may need to start pumping your milk right after your baby is born so you can establish your supply. (Read more about pumping in this chapter.) Seek out expert help. At the hospital, talk to a lactation specialist as soon as possible; she will be in a good position to help protect and support your breastfeeding relationship. Know that providing the best nutrition for your baby is a vital part of his medical care—and surround yourself with people who understand this.

Adoptive Nursing

The word still needs to get out: Women can bring in their own milk supply for an adopted baby (induced lactation); women can also bring back a milk supply after weaning their babies (relactation). All of this usually comes as a surprise to many doctors and nurses, but mothers have done these things. New and better methods for bringing in milk can help mothers attain a full milk supply.

It's true that different women will have different results. A lot depends on the baby's willingness to latch onto the breast and nurse. Yet, those women who have worked at bringing in a milk supply, even if only a few drops, are generally very happy that they tried. These mothers are the first to say that it is hard work and takes a lot of persistence and support—but it's worth it in the end.

There are some excellent publications by La Leche League and the World Health Organization on the topic. (See appendix A.) Some helpful web sites that aim to support the adoptive mother are listed in appendix B as well. Experienced mothers say that nothing is more helpful than reading other women's stories or talking to women about induced lactation or relactation. More and more lactation consultants are familiar with helping mothers breastfeed their adopted children. A number of La Leche League Leaders have breastfed adopted children and can be contacted for tips or help.

Herbs can assist in building or keeping a milk supply. See chapter 7 for more information about low milk supply situations and what to do. You may also find it helpful to consult the book *Ultimate Breastfeeding Book of Answers* by Canadian pediatrician Jack Newman, in which he describes how he uses herbs to help with adoptive nursing. (See appendix A.)

Breastfeeding after Breast Surgery

If you've had any kind of breast surgery, it's worthwhile to learn how that surgery may have affected your ability to breastfeed. The details of the surgery, where cuts were made, and what was removed (breast reduction) or added (breast augmentation) all factor into breastfeeding and any potential problems you may experience.

Each mother-baby pair is unique, so take some time to explore your breastfeeding options. Don't believe it if someone says you "can't" breastfeed because of your surgery. In some cases, it is very possible to breastfeed exclusively after surgery, but some mothers must supplement with formula. However, they can continue to give their babies whatever milk they do make. This is far better for a baby than no milk at all.

La Leche League has published a thorough book on the topic of breastfeeding after breast reduction; the book includes a complete discussion of ways to increase milk supply, which is also good reading for women with other types of breast surgery, adoptive mothers, or anyone else who has a low milk supply. For an introduction to the topic of breastfeeding after surgery, visit the web site of the educational organization Breastfeeding After Reduction: www.bfar.org.

Pumping Your Milk

Working with a breast pump is a learned art. Like breastfeeding itself, pumping takes some time to get accustomed to.

There are many different types of pumps on the market, but, as yet, there are no laws requiring them to meet safety or efficacy standards. Many mothers have found that the cheap battery-operated pumps that are widely available in drugstores aren't very efficient. Such pumps are suitable only if you don't need to pump very often.

However, if your goal is to establish or maintain a full milk supply, you will need a much more efficient pump. For most mothers in this situation, renting a hospital-grade pump with a double hookup (it pumps both breasts at the same time) and an automatic suction-release cycle is the best option. These hospital-grade pumps are very expensive to buy, but they can be rented by the month. If you're separated from your baby or if your baby can't nurse for some reason, look into renting this type of pump; many insurance companies reimburse the rental costs in medical situations.

If you plan to go back to work full-time and want to continue breastfeeding, you may be happy to know that breastfeeding and working aren't mutually exclusive. Many mothers work outside of the home and breastfeed successfully. Working mothers can find a range of less expensive, good quality electric pumps designed with their needs in mind. You can rent or buy these pumps, and the costs vary. There's even a new double pump that fits in your bra, leaving your hands free.

Talk with a lactation specialist about the pros and cons of various electric pumps. You will probably discover that a lactation specialist can help you get started with a pump better than a pharmacy or medical supply store can. La Leche League libraries provide many books and information sheets devoted to the topic of breast pumps, milk storage, and working while breastfeeding. Go to a meeting and talk to mothers who have used pumps. See what they recommend.

🌿 🌿 🌿

No matter what your circumstances, arrange to have supportive voices around you after the birth of your child. Is there someone who can come to your home and prepare meals, do dishes and laundry, or watch the baby while you take a shower or a break? (Think of it as mothering the mother in this special time.) This person's presence can make a big difference, especially if he or she remains supportive of your efforts to breastfeed. The baby's father can be helpful, too, doing double duty as both father and supporter/protector of breastfeeding.

If at any time you have doubts, questions, or thoughts of quitting, reach out to your network of supporters. Find some help. Turn your ear toward those who are knowledgeable and have had a successful experience with breastfeeding. Listen to their suggestions because some of them might work for you. These supporters can help you through the rough spots and keep you going—and they can cheer you on when things go well.

Mother and Baby

The moment your baby is born, your whole world changes. As you hold, nurse, change, and care for your baby in every way, you may start to see him almost as an extension of yourself. Your previous role as an independent woman is temporarily on hold; you become a new person, someone who is completely focused on the baby and his needs. You may gladly dive into a profound relationship with this tiny new person who is totally dependent on you, his mother. Or you may discover that this new relationship is a somewhat difficult, yet manageable, adjustment in your life.

This relationship, in which two people are truly more like one, is intensified through breastfeeding. While nursing, you aren't simply a mother and a baby, but a mother-baby: a *dyad.* The dyad represents a physical connection, an emotional bond, and interdependence. You rely on your baby to take milk from your breasts, relieving them from engorgement and stimulating them to make more milk. Your baby, in turn, depends on your body to make and produce his food. The milk you give him contains not only basic nutrients but a host of other substances that protect him against infections and help his body to develop normally. The physical flow of milk from you to your baby intimately binds the two of you together.

The breastfeeding dyad is only one step removed from the oneness of pregnancy. During pregnancy, substances flow from you to your baby through the placenta. You eat for two, and whatever you consume has consequences for your unborn child. After his birth, the flow of substances continues through your breasts. Entirely dependent on you, your baby consumes whatever milk you make, along with any substances it may contain. You continue eating for two—or at least with two in mind.

Although life changes after you have a child, it's natural to want to eat and drink as others do, and to get your life back in some small way. You may want to have a glass of wine every so often, drink your morning coffee, or eat a bit of chocolate without worrying whether your breastfeeding baby will be harmed. The good news is you don't have to live as a monk in a pure state of being in order to provide healthy milk for your child.

How Milk Is Made and Why This Matters

Every culture has an explanation of where milk comes from. In many traditional societies, it is thought that milk is transformed menstrual blood (because nursing mothers don't menstruate, at least in the first several months after childbirth). The idea isn't that far off target—milk *is* made from transformed substances, the ones nursing mothers consume.

When you eat, your digestive system breaks down food substances into simpler chemical forms. Your liver is the first to receive the chemicals; some of them pass through this organ unchanged and enter your bloodstream. Potentially harmful chemicals are further broken down in your liver, so they can be eliminated from your body. Everything that is destined to be made into milk reaches your breasts through your bloodstream.

But first these chemicals must pass through your milk secretory cells, which serve as a barrier and help manufacture the many unique components of your milk. Breast milk is mostly water, but it also contains the right mix of nutrients and other important substances for your baby. The hundreds of different components in your breast milk are secreted into your milk ducts, where they move down and out of your breasts as you nurse.

How much milk can you count on producing? Generally, three-fourths of a quart to a quart each day. This amount stays surprisingly steady after the first few weeks of breastfeeding until weaning begins. Regardless of what you consume or how often your baby nurses, your milk production will stay remarkably constant from day to day, and from one feeding to the next.

One thing that does change, however, is the proportion of fat in your breast milk. The fat level fluctuates during each breastfeeding session, and from one session to the next. Each time you nurse, your baby gets your thinner foremilk first, followed by the hind milk, which is rich in fat. Your baby needs the hind milk, so it's important to let him nurse long enough at each breast before switching to the other. During each feeding, the taste of your milk may change a bit, too, depending on what you eat or drink. For example, eating fresh garlic will make your milk smell and taste like garlic for a little while.

As a general rule, the substances that get past your liver and into your bloodstream will, most likely, enter your breast milk in small amounts. Certain components of plant foods, for instance, make their way into breast milk: the vitamin C in orange juice, the caffeine in coffee or tea, and the flavonoids that make fruits taste so good. Yet, other plant components, such as bran or fiber, won't enter your breast milk because they stay in your gastrointestinal tract and aren't absorbed into your bloodstream.

Experts are still studying how substances in medicinal plants enter the bloodstream and what effects they have on the body. Research has shown that some elements of medicinal plants remain in the digestive system, never reaching the bloodstream. Other plant elements are immediately broken down in the liver and therefore don't reach the bloodstream, either. What does this mean for a nursing mother? Many ingredients in medicinal plants will never reach your breasts or enter your milk. Those that *do* enter your milk do so in generally tiny amounts. You can rest easier knowing that your breastfeeding baby is naturally protected from receiving large doses of plant chemicals.

But what about over-the-counter medications or prescription drugs? Their entry into breast milk is limited, too. Studies of pharmaceuticals have consistently shown that most medications and prescription drugs do not concentrate in breast milk. As a rule of thumb, about 1 percent of whatever chemical a mother ingests will make it into her breast milk. For most medications and drugs—even powerful ones—this dose is too small to have any measurable effect on the baby. There are exceptions to this rule, so seeking the guidance of a knowledgeable professional is still important.

Knowing that a particular chemical will enter your breast milk is only the beginning. There are specific questions to consider when using medicinal plants, prescription drugs, or other medications while nursing. You may find it helpful to bring the following list of questions when you visit your healthcare provider:

- What is the recommended dose for me, and how much of that dose would my baby consume per day?

- What are the known adverse effects of the substance?

- Could these effects occur from small doses or only in an overdose?

- Are these effects rare or common?

- Are these effects mild and easily reversible, or are they potentially life threatening?

Be sure that your provider is well informed and able to address all of your questions and concerns. For more information about finding knowledgeable healthcare providers, see chapter 5. Consult chapter 4 to learn more about choosing herbal products that are safe.

You and Your Baby Are Unique

Each breastfeeding relationship is one of a kind. So when it comes to the use of foods, herbs, and medicines while nursing, the unique nature of the dyad should be considered. For example, a newborn in the first few weeks of breastfeeding is very different from a toddler who only nurses at night. A mother who is breastfeeding exclusively is different from one who is supplementing with formula. For every mother-baby pair, two initial questions are key: (1) How old is the child? and (2) How often does he nurse?

Yet, most current sources of information about herbs and drugs don't take these questions into account. Instead, they treat all breastfeeding situations as if they were exactly the same. As a nursing mother, you're left with blanket recommendations or warnings for the use of many products. For example, you may read a warning on the label on a dietary supplement or an over-the-counter medication that says the product isn't safe to use while nursing. But the product may not be as dangerous as its label suggests, because what's risky for one nursing pair can be harmless for another. Despite what you may have read or been told by herbal experts or medical professionals, there are many healing plants, herbs, medications, and drugs that are safe for use by nursing mothers.

Before ingesting any medicinal substance, however, take these important factors into account.

Your Child's Age and Weight

Consider your child's age and weight as you and your provider determine how a dose of a substance may affect him. In general, the younger the child the more vulnerable he is, because of his lower body weight and less developed organs.

A newborn's gastrointestinal tract, liver, and kidneys are still immature and therefore are less able to metabolize and eliminate substances. By two weeks of age, a baby's liver is mature, but because his kidneys aren't fully developed until around four months, his ability to eliminate substances is still limited. A six-month-old, on the other hand, has a more mature gastrointestinal tract and is ready for foods other than

Alcohol, Cigarettes, and "Recreational" Drugs

Many mothers wonder whether it's safe to consume any alcohol while breastfeeding. If you drink in moderation, your baby will not be harmed; two alcoholic drinks or less per day have shown no risks to a nursing child. Once your body metabolizes the alcohol and its level in your bloodstream goes down, the alcohol is eliminated from your milk (it doesn't "get stuck there," as some people fear). Interestingly, babies don't care for the taste of pure alcohol, and they tend to nurse less until the alcohol is eliminated. If you regularly abuse alcohol, however, the repercussions for your baby could include slow weight gain or a failure to thrive.

Recreational drugs present a darker picture. Studies have shown that when a mother smokes pot, THC (the active chemical in marijuana) concentrates in her milk and is passed to her breastfeeding baby. THC can be detected in breast milk for many days, and perhaps weeks, after a mother smokes a joint. Because marijuana is an illegal substance, any documented exposure to it in a breastfeeding baby—through a toxicity screen, for example—may be grounds for Child Protection Services to step in. Harder drugs such as heroin or cocaine pose even greater physical risks to breastfeeding babies. Consumption of these drugs through breast milk can cause a baby to become intoxicated or even addicted.

Cigarettes pose risks for babies mostly as a result of *inhalation* of cigarette smoke rather than the consumption of tobacco compounds in breast milk. If you gave up smoking during pregnancy, try not to pick up the habit again. Not only will you stay healthier, but your baby will have the benefit of breathing cleaner air. If needed, chew nicotine gum or use a patch to help quit smoking—the nicotine will break down into another chemical before reaching your breastfeeding baby. If your baby is premature or has other health concerns, talk to your healthcare professional or a breastfeeding expert about the effects smoking may have on him. The bottom line: It's generally considered less risky for a mother to smoke and breastfeed than to wean and feed him baby formula. Remember, however, that inhaling cigarette smoke can harm a child.

breast milk; he can more easily break down substances he ingests. In addition, proteins and other allergens are less likely to "leak" into his bloodstream and cause reactions. (Before six months of age, a baby has a "leaky" gastrointestinal tract, and allergens more easily pass into his blood.) This is why age and weight are so important to consider, especially in the early months of your child's life.

Bear in mind that premature infants, with their tiny bodies and immature organs, are especially vulnerable. For these little ones, expert guidance is needed before using any herb, dietary supplement, medication, or drug.

The Amount of Breast Milk Your Child Consumes

The amount of breast milk your child consumes determines the amount of the medicinal substance he consumes. So, it's important to tell your provider how often your child nurses and whether you're nursing exclusively.

A three-month-old who is breastfeeding exclusively is probably taking in close to a quart of milk each day—but what about a three-month-old who breastfeeds only a couple of times per day and is supplemented with formula? Even if these two babies are the same age and weight, the amount of breast milk they consume is quite different. Similarly, a toddler who nurses only at bedtime probably consumes a small amount of breast milk; one who takes all of his fluids as breast milk, even after the age of two, consumes much more. In general, an infant who is under six months of age and who nurses exclusively consumes the largest amount of breast milk for his weight—and therefore receives the biggest relative dose of substances in the milk.

Your Child's Health

It's important to take special care with a child who has liver, kidney, or digestive problems or any other metabolic condition that makes it harder for him to break down and eliminate chemicals. If your child has health concerns, be sure to let your provider know when you're considering taking any herbs or medications.

Your Own Health Needs

In the past, mothers who needed to take a medication for health reasons were routinely advised to stop breastfeeding. Those who sought herbal treatments instead of medications were told that herbs weren't safe to use while nursing, either. Some were even encouraged to wean if breastfeeding, for whatever reason, wasn't going well. All-or-nothing recommendations like these have forced many mothers to stop breastfeeding or forego health treatments for themselves. Perhaps you've been in a similar situation; if so, you probably wondered if weaning was really the answer.

Because breastfeeding is so important for you and your baby, you're right to question whether weaning is necessary. Why should you have to give up nursing when it's so healthy for you both? Instead of accepting this advice at face value, you can ask your healthcare provider further questions, such as:

- Why, exactly, must I wean?

- What are the benefits of weaning?

- What are the risks of weaning?

- What are the pros and cons of your recommended treatment?

- What other treatment choices are available to me?

- Where is the information to guide us?

It may take time and effort to sort out all of your options and get accurate answers to your questions. But given the importance of breastfeeding, taking the time and effort is well worth it, both for you and your baby.

While weighing your options, keep other important health issues in mind. If you're the mother of a newborn, for example, you may want to avoid any herb that could speed the return of fertility; but, if you're nursing a toddler, you may want to use just such an herb to help you become pregnant again. If you're pregnant and nursing a toddler, you'll need to avoid herbs that stimulate uterine activity (so you don't go into premature labor). If you have a particular health problem, such as poor liver or kidney function, it's best to know which medicinal agents are risky for your condition so you can avoid them. And if you have allergies or food sensitivities, you'll need to take precautions with substances that may trigger a reaction in either you or your baby. Appendix C is a good starting point for learning about the relative safety of specific herbs.

Knowing that certain herbs can affect the amount of milk you produce is important as well. Some herbs will increase your milk supply, while others will slow it down. If you're happy with your milk supply, you may want to avoid ingesting substances that could alter it in some way. Read more about herbs that affect milk supply in chapter 7.

❦ ❦ ❦

As a nursing mother, you're making decisions for two, which means you must always take both your needs and your child's into account. But it is possible to strike a balance. Few medicinal substances are strictly off-limits. Even prescription drugs are generally compatible with breastfeeding. Yet safety is a relative thing. Is the treatment safe or unsafe—compared to what? To weaning and formula? To using another drug or herb? These are the pertinent questions. While nobody can guarantee that a particular drug or herb will be absolutely safe for you to use, in most cases you and your healthcare provider can determine if it may be safer or riskier than other treatment options.

When it comes to your health, always remember that you have a right and a responsibility to ask questions of your healthcare provider and to share your own knowledge with him or her. After all, *you* know your baby, yourself, and your circumstances better than anyone else. And in the end, it is you who must decide what is truly best for you both.

Herbs and Herbal Products

BECOMING A KNOWLEDGEABLE CONSUMER

These days, there always seems to be some new "wonder" product on the market, promising to solve your every health concern. It can be confusing to choose from the array of products available from drugstores, health-food stores, and the Internet. You may wonder if these products are as safe, reliable, and effective as they claim.

How can you as a consumer find answers to your questions about the herbs and herbal products you see on store shelves, in magazine ads, or on television? First, you need to understand how herbs are classified in comparison to prescription drugs, over-the-counter (OTC) medications, and other kinds of dietary supplements.

Prescription drugs require a doctor's permission to use because they have great potential for harm when used inappropriately. A doctor decides the type of drug to prescribe and the best dose for the patient, then instructs the patient on use of the drug. Over-the-counter

Note: The information in this chapter reflects current regulation of food and drugs in the United States. Herbal regulations in other countries may vary.

medications, on the other hand, have been shown to be safe for general consumers to use on their own—in other words, to self-prescribe their use. These medications are freely available for purchase. Consumers who buy these products are expected to use them appropriately, which means taking responsibility for reading and following the instructions printed on the labels. Both prescription drugs and OTC medications are made to specific pharmaceutical standards.

Dietary supplements are a type of over-the-counter product that consumers can buy freely. These natural compounds are consumed in addition to food but aren't actually considered food (at least in the regulatory sense). In the United States, the term "dietary supplement" is based on a legal definition, rather than a medicinal or nutritional one. Dietary supplements are regulated like food in how they are manufactured, but they differ from food in that they require special labeling about their health claims.

All herbal products in nonfood forms are regulated as dietary supplements, as are vitamin and mineral supplements. Some foods are also considered medicinal herbs and are sold as both a food and a supplement. (Garlic, for example, is offered as a food in fresh bulbs and as a dietary supplement in the form of pills.) These days, many new "hybrid" food products have had various herbs, vitamins, minerals, and other natural substances added to them in small amounts.

Confused? Many people are, and it's easy to see why. Foods and medicines can't always be sharply divided into two separate categories, so the line between them is blurry. The legal term "dietary supplement" attempts to straddle this line. In the United States, products sold as food will have "nutrition facts" on the label, while those sold as dietary supplements will have "supplement facts" on the label. (In comparison, OTC medicines list "active ingredients" and "indications for use" on the label.)

As you can see, it's not always easy to know what you're buying and how to use each product appropriately.

Using Herbs Safely

Contrary to an often-repeated misconception, the American herbal industry is regulated by the Food and Drug Administration (FDA). All herbal products and other dietary supplements must be manufactured according to food-production standards in the United States. As with foods, their labels are required to identify all of the products' contents and to be free of contamination. Herbal products that are sold in the U.S. must not contain herbs that have been banned due to toxicity. The FDA monitors all herbs of commerce for toxicity and other problems.

Most herbs for sale in the United States have undergone government safety reviews. The majority of the herbs available here are GRAS (generally regarded as safe); however, a few popular ones are not. GRAS status isn't required for dietary supplements, though manufacturers can apply for GRAS status if they want to.

Few herbs have been proven toxic, and those that have cannot be sold legally in the United States. Yet, in many other parts of the world, truly unregulated herb markets still exist. Occasionally, products containing toxic herbs are imported from abroad; the FDA seizes and removes them when found.

Still, the FDA's monitoring system for herbal products isn't as extensive or well funded as the one for OTC or prescription medications. For example, the FDA doesn't require herb companies to automatically report when a consumer has experienced adverse effects from an herbal product. However, they are required to keep records of any adverse reactions and produce the documents if asked to do so by the government. Because the FDA's product-monitoring programs lack the funds to hire enough inspectors to do a thorough job, the threat of contamination or misidentification of herbal products is an ongoing concern. To confuse matters, the labels on herbal products aren't always reliable and may not provide enough information for consumers. When herbs are sold in bulk, they may not be labeled at all.

As a consumer, you have the right to use the herbal products of your choice, but it's your responsibility to use these herbal products safely. A handful of commercial herbs remain controversial and are considered by the Food and Drug Administration to be of "undetermined safety." These herbs do have legitimate uses in herbal medicine and haven't been proven dangerous, as long as they're used properly. The Dietary Supplement Health and Education Act, which ensures that consumers have freedom of access to herbs and other dietary supplements, restrains the FDA from unnecessarily removing useful but potentially risky herbs when toxicity hasn't been proven.

Such is the case with the herb ephedra. This herb is a stimulant that can cause serious problems, especially when taken in large doses and combined with other stimulant herbs. (Because such use is potentially dangerous, it is viewed by experts as being completely inappropriate.) Ephedra has been shown to be useful for the treatment of asthma when used for a short time in small doses—a use that dates back many thousands of years in China. Consumers who use ephedra for weight loss, on the other hand, may be putting themselves at risk because most weight-loss products with ephedra also contain caffeine, a potentially dangerous combination. Almost all adverse incidents involving ephedra have been a result of consumers using ephedra-caffeine combination products. (Read more about ephedra in chapter 9.)

Herbs, like ephedra, that have clear safety concerns require considerably more caution and may not be safe for some people. But this can also be said of many OTC medications. For example, acetaminophen is a medication that can be found in any drugstore; yet, overdoses can be deadly, and people who have liver problems shouldn't use products containing this substance. About two hundred cases of liver toxicity occur every year in the U.S. from acetaminophen taken at recommended dosages. Although OTC medications are approved for self-use, they must be taken carefully. Herbs have to be used carefully, too. However, very few herbs sold commercially have been shown to have the potentially serious side effects of OTC medications.

Safe use of herbs requires knowledge of (1) the herb itself and (2) the herbal product. There is a difference between the two. An herb's safety depends on the nature of the plant and its effects, but the safety of an herbal product depends on many things, including how it was manufactured. In other words, a perfectly safe herb can be made into an unsafe product whose effects have nothing to do with the plant itself.

Understanding the Herb

This book cannot tell you everything you need to know about each and every herb, but it can give you a good place to start. See appendix A for a helpful list of other reliable herb books—general herbals, women's herbals, and reference texts—that you can consult. Many herbalists have access to even more detailed reference texts; health-food stores may have them, too. Be aware that many books and articles will likely recommend avoiding the use of herbs during breastfeeding. These recommendations don't have to be taken at face value, though. (Review chapter 3, which discusses how breast milk is made and what substances enter into the milk.) When in doubt, talk to a breastfeeding expert or an herbal helper before using herbs.

As you begin your research, keep in mind that current knowledge of a particular herb is based on the properties of a high-quality plant—and not all plants are grown or preserved equally well. The full benefits cannot be derived from a plant that has crumbled into dust, for example. The best way to learn about an herb is to find a way to meet the living-plant. If possible, grow, harvest, and preserve plants yourself. Or find someone in your community who knows herbs and plants. This person may offer courses on making herbal preparations or hold "plant walks" at local nature centers, giving you the chance to see, smell, touch, and taste the herb.

Become familiar with each herb's botanical name. An herb can have many common names but only one botanical name.* Botanical names are written in Latin and have a capitalized first name (the genus) and a

---

* Some common names are quite similar to their botanical names. For example, ginkgo is *Ginkgo biloba,* and echinacea refers to one of three *Echinacea* species used medicinally. But most common names differ significantly from their botanical names. For example, the plant known by the common name nettle (or stinging nettle) has the botanical name *Urtica dioica.*

lowercase second name (the species). Garlic is *Allium sativum,* onion is *Allium cepa,* and chives are *Allium schoenoprasum.* Learning the Latin names may seem difficult, but it's worth the effort. When you know the botanical name and its proper spelling, you can look up the herb in a reference book or ask an expert about it with less confusion.

While it may seem obvious, you'll need to learn what the herb is used for and whether it is appropriate for your particular situation. Consider such questions such as: How can the herb help? Is it appropriate for this particular health issue? What other herbs might help, and do they appear safer? Is an herb the best response, or is it better to use a medication? Is it possible to fix the problem without the use of herbs or medicines? For example, would diet and exercise help as much?

Learn exactly how the particular herb or plant is used. Is it taken internally (by mouth) or externally (on the skin)? Is it safe to use on mucous membranes or open skin? Many herbs that aren't safe to take internally shouldn't be applied to open wounds, either. Arnica, for example, is toxic if taken internally or put on open skin; yet, it is perfectly safe when applied to help heal bruises, if the skin is intact.

Find out which part of the plant is being used and for what purpose. Sometimes, the fruit of the plant is used for one thing, but the root is used for something else. For example, the fruit of the blackberry is considered a healthful food, while the root bark is used medicinally for diarrhea. In

A Note of Caution

If you're using herbs that you or someone else has collected in the wild, or even from a garden, make sure you have the right plant. Some toxic plants look very similar to herbs, so always be careful.

some cases, one part of the plant may be eaten, but another part may be toxic. Bilberry fruit, for instance, makes both a delicious jam and a useful medicine, but the leaves are potentially toxic. For a few herbs, the fresh plant is never used, since only dried preparations are safe.

One of the most important things to know about an herb is what constitutes a safe dose. The amount you take can determine whether the herb helps or, in some cases, harms you. Find out what a typical dose is, and don't exceed it unless you're specifically guided to do so by an expert herbal practitioner who also understands your breastfeeding situation. If you're looking at an herbal product label, make sure the dose on the label agrees with the information you already have.

In general, whenever you use an herb follow the rule of thumb recommended for medications: Choose the lowest dose that will be effective and use it for only as long as necessary. If you're using an herb continuously for preventive purposes, use the most benign herb available and take a break from using it for a few days every couple of weeks.

Acquaint yourself with any known side effects that an herb may cause. A number of herbs cause side effects such as nausea, vomiting, or diarrhea. If you experience these effects, you might try a lower dose or even avoiding the herb for a day or two before trying it again at a lower dose. Be aware that your body simply may not agree with a particular herb, for whatever reason. Try using another one, if desired. Always respect your own body's response to a particular herb.

Choose herbs that have mild and "reversible" side effects, so they won't cause permanent harm. Steer clear of herbs that are known to have severe or dangerous side effects. When breastfeeding, it may be best to avoid those herbs that can cause side effects even in small doses; instead, find herbs with a wider margin of safety. And never use toxic plants—those with severe and irreversible side effects. If a book you're consulting doesn't discuss an herb's known side effects, consult another source or talk to an expert you trust.

People with certain conditions should not use certain herbs. Some herbs are known allergens. (See the previous page for more on allergies.) Others have effects that aren't safe for people with particular medical

Herbs and Allergies

If either you or the father of your child has a family history of allergies, eczema, asthma, insulin-dependent diabetes, and rheumatoid arthritis or other autoimmune diseases, you need to be especially cautious about certain foods and herbs. Others may wish to minimize their chances of an allergic reaction as well.

Three medicinal plant families are well known for their allergic potential: the Fabaceae, or pea family; the Asteraceae, or sunflower family; and the Apiaceae, or carrot family. Soy and peanuts are common plants in the pea family, and herbs such as fenugreek, goat's rue, and licorice are also members of this family. Members of the carrot family include carrots, parsnips, and celery; common herbs in this family are celery seed, anise, and fennel. People can be sensitive to the essential oil in all of these seeds. You may want to be cautious with plants such as chamomile and possibly echinacea as well, as both are related to ragweed, which is known to be a major cause of hay fever. But echinacea has not been directly linked to allergy, and chamomile has only very rarely caused allergic reactions (with most cases involving Roman, not German, chamomile). Other members of this family, including mugwort and elecampane, are well-known allergens. Members of the citrus family can also trigger allergic reactions, as can tree nuts, wheat, and corn. See appendix C for more information on the allergic potential of common herbs.

problems. For example, licorice is known to increase blood pressure in high doses and therefore isn't recommended for people who already have high blood pressure. Some herbs contain plant chemicals that can affect major organs such as the kidneys, liver, and heart. Uva-ursi, for example, is mildly irritating to the kidneys; although it may be fairly safe for healthy people, it clearly shouldn't be used by someone with a kidney problem.

Some herbs may have unexpected effects on your milk supply or fertility. Before using an herb for any purpose, try to learn whether it is also used to increase or decrease a mother's milk supply, or to affect her fertility. In addition, many herbs should be avoided or used with great care during pregnancy, as they may cause premature labor. Chapter 7 has information on herbs and milk supply; chapter 11 discusses herbs and fertility. I encourage you to read through these sections and consult a lactation specialist for more information about your situation.

It's important to know whether any other herbs, foods, over-the-counter medications, or prescription drugs will interact with the herb you wish to use. Some herbs are known to increase or decrease the effects of other medicines. Often, this interaction is only significant when high doses of the herb are used. If you're taking prescription or OTC drugs, you need to pay special attention to any known interactions with herbs. Always seek guidance from those who are knowledgeable about your medical care and about the herb in question.

One final consideration: Is the plant endangered as a result of over-harvesting? Some widely used plants are near extinction in the wild, even though alternative crop plants could and should be used. See Rosemary Gladstar's books for more information on this topic; you'll find a listing of her books in appendix A.

Appendix C rates herbs according to known safety issues. You can consult the ratings to find out which herbs are safer for self-use and which ones require more information or a consultation before use. Some herbs in the list should be avoided entirely, as they're not worth the risk while breastfeeding. All of the herbs in appendix C are rated with the nursing mother in mind. Known allergens, as well as herbs that are used to increase or decrease milk supply, are also clearly identified.

Despite all the concerns I've brought up here, please do not get the impression that herbs are dangerous. As a group, herbs are probably safer than most other types of medications. Many herbs have no known safety concerns, and many more are safe for most people to use. Herbs generally cause few side effects, and only rarely are these side effects judged to be serious or permanent. Very few medicinal plants sold in the United States are inherently dangerous. Most serious safety concerns derive from the risks of improper handling and packaging: misidentified plants, contamination, or dangerous combinations.

But because some herbs do carry risks, you need to do your homework before using a new herb. Whenever an herb has potential safety concerns, consult with your healthcare provider before use. Similarly, if the label on a particular herb or herbal product recommends consulting a healthcare provider, be sure to do so. And you should definitely consult your doctor if you're receiving treatment for an illness or taking medications. See chapter 5 for more information about talking with healthcare providers.

Understanding the Herbal Product

Once you have learned about an herb, there still remains the question of which herbal products are the best and safest for use. Herbs can be prepared in many forms: teas, decoctions, tinctures, capsules, concentrates, and essential oils, to name a few. Herbal preparations or products differ in how, and how well, they work; in some cases, they may present different safety considerations. Understanding what the various herbal terms mean can help you choose wisely from the many preparations on the market.

You can make your own herbal preparations using fresh or dried herbs—a wonderful way to learn about and connect with plants. The traditional methods of preparing herbs in teas or tinctures are simple and inexpensive. A basic herb book will usually include a section on making herbal products at home. (For recommended books, see appendix A.) Chapter 7 contains a brief introduction to the ancient art of making herbal preparations, as well as more detailed instructions for making galactogogue teas (those that increase milk supply).

Herbal preparations are of two basic types: "simples," which contain a single herb, and mixtures, which contain more than one herb. An herb used for a particular health condition is considered a "specific" for that condition and is traditionally used alone (i.e., as a simple). Simple herbal products are advantageous for nursing mothers. If there is a reaction with you or your baby, it is easy to identify the culprit. However, if you react to a product that is a mixture of different herbs, it will be much harder to know which plant is causing the ill effect.

And yet, many traditional recipes, such as Chinese medicinal remedies, often contain a number of different herbs that have been found to work well together or to work better than simples. (Typically, about five to seven herbs make up the recipes.) These mixtures usually contain smaller quantities of any single herb as compared to a simple, which decreases the likelihood of dose-related side effects. Traditional recipes have the advantage of having stood the test of time; their effects and side effects are known and are therefore more predictable than new combinations. Some traditional recipes and herbals are easily made at home; see chapter 7 for ideas and instructions.

Some modern herb products list a large number of ingredients on their labels. On some products you may see lists of vitamins and minerals, and perhaps a number of isolated plant constituents, along with several herbs in suspiciously tiny doses. These long, impressive-looking lists are probably not time-tested, traditional recipes. Be aware that a long list of ingredients doesn't necessarily indicate a superior mixture or product. When in doubt, ask an herbal practitioner for guidance.

Common Herbal Products

In the following pages, you'll find a list of some common herbal forms you may have heard about. These preparations all start with the whole herb, and the finished product contains a wide range of the chemicals found in the original plant. Plant chemicals differ in how well they are extracted in water, alcohol, or other solvents. For this reason, different ways of preparing herbs have been developed over the years. The common forms discussed here have been in use for over a millennium. (Note that these preparations may be made as simples or mixtures, and that some herbal products combine preparation methods.)

Teas (also known as tisanes or infusions): An infusion is prepared using dried plant material that's covered with boiling water in a teacup or pot, then steeped for a short period of time. You can easily make teas and tea blends starting with dried bulk herbs. Tea bags are a convenience, but the herbs may quickly degrade if they aren't stored properly. Some aromatic seeds such as fennel need to be crushed just before use; their properties are not well extracted in a tea bag.

Decoctions: Dried plant materials—often the heavier plant parts, like roots—are added to cold water and brought to a boil, then simmered for a long time (sometimes hours) to extract their properties. You will not see ready-made decoctions in stores; they are prepared at home from bulk herbs.

Liquid extracts: These products start with the "crude" herb (whole plant or plant part) soaked in various liquids (water, alcohol, glycerin, or mixtures of these). The resulting liquid is separated out from the insoluble parts. Liquid extracts prepared with water-alcohol mixtures are commonly called tinctures. For some herbs (like oat straw), glycerin is preferred for use in making the liquid extract; these products are called glycerites.

Commercial liquid extracts usually state on the label the ratio of plant material to fluid that is used to make the extract. One of the advantages of liquid extracts is that a dose is usually only a few drops. Commercial liquid extracts may be variously concentrated, so follow the dose recommendation for each product.

When a 1:1 (or 1:2) ratio of plant material to water is used to make a liquid extract, the resulting product is called a fluidextract (e.g., 1 gram of plant material is used to make 1 milliliter of fluid). Some fluidextract products are made by reconstituting dried concentrated plant extracts. Fluidextracts are more concentrated than tinctures (see below), as tinctures are usually made at a 1:5 ratio. Note that most liquid extracts in American stores are tinctures, though you may sometimes see fluidextracts, too.

Tinctures or alcoholic extracts: Tinctures are herb preparations that use alcohol with water to make a fairly dilute liquid extract. (Using a mixture of alcohol and water extracts a wider range of plant chemicals than water alone.) For some herbs, a tincture extract simply works better.

When making a tincture, plant material is chopped and covered with a mixture of water and alcohol, then allowed to steep so the plant chemicals can leach into the liquid. The liquid is bottled afterwards. To do this at home, you'll most likely need fresh plant materials, but this depends on the herb. (A few herbs can be used dried.) Brandy and vodka both contain an effective mixture of ethanol and water for extracting most herbs. Commercial tinctures may use more concentrated ethanol mixtures, depending on their purposes. Tinctures can keep for years if stored properly. (They must be well sealed and placed away from heat and light.) Dried herbs, on the other hand, quickly deteriorate and have a limited shelf life even under the best storage conditions.

Store-bought tinctures should have a statement that tells you how much plant material was used per volume of water and alcohol. This ratio is often a 1:5, a 1:6, or even a 1:7 plant-alcohol mixture, but this can vary from product to product. (A ratio of 1:5 means that 1 g of plant material was used to make 5 mL of tincture.) The dose statement allows a rough comparison of tincture doses to whole-herb preparations. Some tincture labels give the dose in terms of your body weight. However, the way the manufacturer makes the product greatly influences the effective dose, so be sure to follow the recommendations on the label.

If you wish to avoid alcohol, you can choose nonalcoholic liquid extracts like glycerites, or use dried extract forms (such as pills and capsules). Or you can put the tincture drops into a cup of warm water and let the mixture sit until the alcohol evaporates off and can no longer be smelled. (The alcohol content in a tincture may look high, but only a few drops are taken at a time. Some have said there is more alcohol in a ripe banana than in a typical tincture dose.)

Pills and capsules: Although you can fill capsules at home from bulk powdered herbs, most people tend to purchase herbs in pills or capsules for convenience. People who dislike the taste of some herbs in liquid form may use pills or capsules as well. Echinacea, for example, may taste simply horrible as a tea or tincture, and capsules of this dried herb tend to be more tolerable on the taste buds. (On the other hand, the bad taste of some herbs is thought to stimulate the glands of the gastrointestinal tract, giving you more benefit. And you certainly learn more about the plant when you taste it.)

When herbs are sold in the form of a pill or capsule, it's more difficult to tell whether they contain high-quality herbs or stale powder. This is especially true when trying to compare capsules that contain the "crude" herb, which is simply dried and powdered. Many dried extracts of an herb come in pill and capsule forms. They have been made in a very specific way and are somewhat more concentrated than a liquid extract. (Often, a 4:1 ratio is used.) Such products may be more expensive, but they're usually of high quality and tend to keep better.

Simple powdered herb capsules are less concentrated than dried extracts in capsules, which is why it's important to follow the dose on each product's label. For example, you would need to take four 250 mg capsules of a simple powdered herb product to get a dose of 1 g of the dried herb. However, you would need to take only one 250 mg capsule of a solid extract product labeled 4:1 to get the equivalent amount of the herb (because the extract is four times as concentrated as the original whole herb). If this seems confusing, keep in mind that the manufacturer will have worked this out already on the label's recommended dose.

Do not assume that all capsules of an herb are the same strength. Capsules come in different sizes: 200, 350, and even 600 mg sizes are common. You may read "Take 2 capsules," but what is the weight of the capsule? And are the capsules filled with a powdered herb or the more concentrated extract? You need to be very clear on the answers to these questions, as this will determine the dose you'll receive.

Concentrates: A concentrated herbal product is one in which large amounts of raw plant material are reduced to a much smaller final product. While herbalists have long made extracts that are somewhat concentrated (e.g., fluidextracts, tinctures), modern technology can now create highly concentrated herbal products that may have new and useful properties.

An example of a new highly concentrated product is ginkgo; 40 to 50 lbs. of ginkgo leaves make 1 lb. of ginkgo concentrate. Ginkgo is concentrated using an extraction process that removes allergenic compounds along with the more inactive parts of the leaf, while concentrating the active ingredients. Although a simple tea can be made with the leaf, this preparation hasn't been shown to effectively improve memory. Highly concentrated ginkgo, on the other hand, has been shown to slow down the development of dementia.

Traditional herbalists often recommend against the use of highly concentrated products, because many of the plant constituents are removed, leaving high amounts of only a few select constituents. Also, the new, highly concentrated products don't have the benefit of traditional wisdom and experience to back them up. While it's true that many of these new products have been scientifically researched, the studies don't include breastfeeding women (or pregnant women or children, for that matter). Even though some of these highly concentrated products appear to be relatively safe, others may have problems that researchers are, as yet, unaware of. As a nursing mother, it is wise to view highly concentrated products with caution; older and more traditional preparations may be safer.

Essential oils: The alchemists of antiquity, who sought the essential nature of each plant, first developed these oils when they invented distillation. They learned to separate the water, alcohol, and other parts of aromatic plants, leaving behind only the fragrant, oily essence of the plant. Most essential oils are still made by distilling the volatile plant oils from an alcoholic extract.

Essential oils smell like the fresh plant material they're derived from, but because they're so highly concentrated, they can have very different properties. For this reason, it's best to use essential oils with care. Remember, it may take hundreds of pounds of flowers to make a pound of essential oil, and this oil contains only the volatile part of the plant. A large body of traditional information exists about essential oils, as they've been used for hundreds and hundreds of years. It is vital to be informed about any essential oil you're interested in using.

Most essential oils, with a few exceptions, aren't intended for internal use; many are toxic if consumed. External use usually requires proper dilution in neutral oils, such as olive oil, to prevent skin irritation. Some essential oils are allergenic and may cause a rash. A few essential oils shouldn't be used anywhere near the face of an infant or a toddler, as they can cause breathing problems. (See chapter 10 for more on keeping your child safe.) Essential oils are powerful agents and always need to be treated with caution in their undiluted state. But when properly used, essential oils can provide a profound benefit for the mind and body, while delighting the senses.

Before using any essential oil, even externally, it is absolutely necessary to learn whether it may be toxic, irritating, or allergenic. And you need to know the dose recommendations, too. For example, how diluted should an external preparation actually be? And if the essential oil is used internally, how many drops can be taken? See "Aromatherapy" in chapter 5 for more on this topic.

Note that essential oils are different from infusion oils, which are simply neutral oils that have had herbs soaked in them. Herbal infusion oils such as arnica oil or St. John's wort oil should not be confused with the much more concentrated essential oils.

Products That Don't Qualify as Herbals Products

There are many dietary supplements to choose from, and not all are herbal products. Only those products that are derived solely from plants can be considered herbal products. Dietary supplements such as vitamins, minerals, animal products, or those containing single plant chemicals (plant isolates) are not herbal products. Even though isolates are derived from plants, they are more like pharmaceuticals than herbs. (See discussion below.) Similarly, health products known as homeopathics and flower essences don't qualify as herbal products. While most homeopathics and flower essences begin with the whole plant, the finished products contain very little actual plant material. These products are often confused with herbals, so it's important for consumers to understand how and why they differ.

Isolates: For almost two hundred years, medical researchers have extracted single chemicals from plants in order to make more powerful medicines. The chemical morphine, for example, is extracted from opium poppy latex; it is then purified so that it may be used in medicine in the precise doses needed. Today, some companies in the herbal industry extract plant chemicals such as lycopene from tomatoes and then sell the chemicals in the form of a pricey pill. (That's one expensive way to get lycopene, a chemical that occurs naturally in tomatoes. Herb author and expert James Duke would probably ask, "Why not just eat lots of tomatoes?") The truth is, when you eat tomatoes, you not only get lycopene but all of the other good chemicals that are found in tomatoes as well. Why settle for just one plant chemical in a pill when hundreds are available in the whole plant?

In addition, an isolate may have more side effects than the herb it's derived from. The natural mixture of chemicals in a whole plant is thought to balance out the harsher effects of one isolated chemical. This is the safety advantage of herbs over isolates: fewer, milder side effects. Some manufacturers add isolates to make their products more impressive to consumers who may believe "more is better" or think they're getting more for the money. But there is no traditional or scientific knowledge to prove that this is always a safe thing to do. According to many herbalists, the safest way to take herbs is in their natural form, or as close to it as possible. To get all of the health benefits that healing plants have to offer, look for foods and herbs in their naturally complex state. Whenever possible, choose whole foods and simpler, gentler herbs.

Nutraceuticals: Nutraceuticals can be broadly defined as naturally occurring components of food or medicinal plants, animal products, and vitamins and minerals that are thought to have therapeutic effects. A nutraceutical is generally taken in amounts much greater than what would normally be consumed as part of the human diet. Herbal products are often included in the definition of nutraceutical, but in this book "nutraceutical" is a shorthand term referring to the host of other dietary supplements that are not herbs.

Like pharmaceuticals, many nutraceuticals contain only one chemical as an ingredient. Plus, nutraceuticals tend to be expensive. It's debatable whether these products are truly worth the money, though in some cases they may be.

Following are some of the nutraceuticals currently available:

- Among the vitamin and mineral products are the "high-potency" or "megadose" products containing perhaps a thousand times more of a vitamin or mineral than is found in a normal diet.

- Some nutraceutical products are isolates derived from herbs. Well-known examples include bromelain from pineapple, isoflavones from soybeans, and Pycnogenol from the maritime pine tree.

- Therapeutic substances from animals include glucosamine from the shells (chitin) of shrimp and lobster, shark cartilage, and purified DHA from fish oils.

- Some compounds in nutraceuticals are hormones (melatonin, for example) or are hormone-containing extracts (such as adrenal extracts from cows).

Are nutraceuticals safe? Some are believed to be quite safe, while others may be questionable. It simply isn't possible to generalize, other than to say that nursing mothers should use caution when considering nutraceuticals. Unlike most herbs, nutraceutical products haven't been fully established as safe by either traditional knowledge or scientific study. Many nutraceuticals are new formulations of old products; other nutraceuticals are just fancy-sounding descriptions of nothing special. However, it must be said that some nutraceuticals truly are new or improved products that hold great promise for improving health.

While lactation experts are still learning about many of the new nutraceuticals, much is already known about the use of vitamins and minerals during breastfeeding. As a nursing mother, it's wise to avoid high-dose vitamins, especially fat-soluble vitamins like A, D, and E. Research has also shown that it's a good idea to avoid sky-high doses of minerals. You can read more about vitamins and minerals in the breastfeeding books listed in appendix A.

Even if a healthcare provider suggests that a nutraceutical product may help you, it's a good idea to also seek out a lactation specialist who may have additional information to guide you. (There is very little information on most new products, however.)

Homeopathics: Many homeopathic products are made starting with a plant extract, but the similarities to herbal products end there. (Chapter 5 includes a discussion of homeopathy.)

Although homeopathic remedies are generally considered safe, many of the substances used in them are deadly poisons: arsenic; heavy metals such as mercury and lead; and highly toxic plants such as belladonna, aconite (monkshood), pokeweed, and arnica. In the making of the homeopathic remedy, these substances are diluted so much that they may not be materially present in the final form. However, because the starting materials are often toxic, the Food and Drug Administration regulates homeopathic remedies as drugs, and they are manufactured according to strict pharmaceutical standards. Reputable homeopathic substances should be labeled HPUS (Homeopathic Pharmacopoeia of the United States) or should include an NDC (National Drug Code) number. Products with these labels have been made according to validated homeopathic procedures that ensure safety.

Flower essences: In the 1920s, Edward Bach began to use flower essences for healing. He floated flowers in water under sunlight, collected the water after several hours, and studied how his emotions were affected when he drank it. He developed a large number of preparations for various emotional states. His most famous preparation is a combination product he called Rescue

A Note of Caution

Homeopathic remedies are named for the substance from which they were made. Many are made from a plant, starting with an herbal tincture (mother tincture) or other standard herbal extract, which is then diluted to make the homeopathic preparation. It's important not to confuse a tincture with a homeopathic remedy. For example, arnica tincture may be placed on the store shelf near the homeopathic remedy, Arnica. There is a difference between the products, however. Arnica tincture is dangerous when used internally; homeopathic Arnica is not. Whenever you're reading about herbal or homeopathic remedies, check to make sure that the distinction between them is clear. Appendix C lists many herbs that are available as homeopathic remedies. In homeopathic form they may be safe, but in an herbal preparation they may be dangerous.

Remedy. Bach believed that his remedies would offer people the gentle nudge needed to regain a healthy state.

In recent years, a number of companies have started making flower essences in the manner of Bach. If you're interested in purchasing products made from flower essences, please note that they do not contain essential oils; essential oils are made by distilling plants with alcohol to extract their pure essence. (See "Essential oils" in this chapter for more on this process.) The Bach approach to extracting a flower's essential nature is the ultimate in gentleness, using only the sun's rays and pure water. They are extremely dilute extracts; a small amount of alcohol is used as a preservative. Be sure that the flower essence products you purchase are exactly that, and not essential oils.

The Quality of Herbal Products

If you're concerned about the quality of the herbal products you buy (and who isn't?), you can look for those that are standardized. Herbs that have been well researched are more likely to be available in standardized forms, which simply means that the product contains plant material with a guaranteed amount of a particular plant chemical. This standard, or marker, chemical is a natural ingredient of the plant, and the amount listed on the label of the packaged herbal product is what that plant is known to contain under natural growing conditions. However, just as crops of wine grapes vary in taste from year to year depending on growing conditions, crops of herbs vary in the amount of plant chemicals they contain. The manufacturer of a standardized herbal product blends many batches of plant material so that the marker chemical is evened out as much as possible.

A standardized herbal product can, however, be badly made if a small amount of high-quality plant material is mixed with a large amount of poor material. Although the final mix may contain the right amount of the marker chemical, other beneficial chemicals found in the high-quality herb may be reduced. This is like making coffee with a small amount of rich coffee beans mixed with a lot of cheap decaffeinated beans. The end product might have the desired amount of caffeine, but it probably won't taste very good. As coffee drinkers know, there's more to coffee than the caffeine; good coffee contains a host of flavorful plant chemicals found only in beans of high quality. The same is true for herbs. The marker chemical may or may not be the only one that makes the herb helpful. Plant scientists are always finding out new explanations for an herb's effects.

A true standardized product will have a statement on the label indicating how much of a particular plant chemical is in each pill or capsule. This statement assures consumers that the maker of the product carefully examined the plant materials that were used. The main advantage of standardization is that it's a good indicator of quality. Companies that go to the trouble of standardizing their products are also likely to check them for bacterial or fungal contamination. This is especially true for products made in Germany, where many rules govern how a plant extract is standardized. The government enforces these rules by closely monitoring herb manufacturers. Of course, you pay a lot more for this oversight.

For many herbs, no standard has yet been developed. This doesn't mean the herb is inferior—only that it hasn't been as well researched or isn't as widely popular (at least for now). A good way to determine the quality of herbal products—whether standardized or not—is to look at the information on their labels, which can tell you a lot about the manufacturers' quality-control practices.

Always check to make sure that a product label contains the following information:

The herb's botanical name: An herbal product should list the botanical names of all the plants used to make it. If the scientific name for a plant isn't there, the manufacturer may not be very sophisticated, which can be a warning sign. If possible, check to see if the botanical names are spelled correctly. You can use appendix C to look up the spellings of botanical names, or check other herbal reference books, if needed. Some herbal products list apothecary names instead, which is acceptable, too. Apothecary names often look like botanical names. (For example, the herb rosemary,

Rosmarinus officinalis, has the apothecary name *Rosmarini folium,* indicating that the leaf of the plant was used to make the product.)

The dose: The dose should be clearly identified. For capsules and pills, the dose includes how many pills or capsules to take at a time, and how many times per day. The weight of each capsule or pill should be listed in milligrams (mg) or grams (g). For liquid forms of an herbal product, the number of drops or the amount in a dropper should be spelled out. The label should also indicate the amount of plant material that went into making each volume of fluid. No matter which form of the product you choose, there should be enough information on the label for you to figure out the recommended maximum dose per day.

An FDA disclaimer statement: Labels usually contain information about what the product can be used for, often in the form of a carefully worded statement about how the herb "supports" the healthy functioning of the mind or body. When you see this, you should also be able to find the following disclaimer: "This statement has not been evaluated by the FDA. This product is not intended to treat, cure, or prevent any disease." Products that claim to do more than support healthy functioning may be overstating what they can do. If the product doesn't include the above FDA disclaimer, its maker is probably a company that doesn't know or follow the FDA rules. (What other rules, then, may the company be disregarding?)

The manufacturer's name and contact information: There should be a street address, phone number, and/or web site address to contact if you have any questions, concerns, or problems. If you do contact the company, the people there should seem happy to hear from you and be willing to answer questions and provide information. If the people you speak with are evasive, poorly informed, or grumpy, you have a right to be skeptical about the quality of their products.

An expiration date: It's important to know when the product is due to expire, or lose its effectiveness. (Lot numbers help responsible manufacturers identify problems with the batches they produce, so look for these numbers, too.)

Quality-control references: Check for information about the company's quality-control standards, or details about its manufacturing process. No single "seal of approval" is in wide use yet, but the following seals of quality are coming into use: the USP (United States Pharmacopoeia) seal of approval and the NSF (formerly known as the National Sanitary Foundation) international seal. These seals mean that the product has been made according to good manufacturing processes (GMPs) but don't actually guarantee that it is safe or effective. You may even see the initials "USP" used without the seal; this is deceiving because the manufacturer is claiming that the ingredients used in the product meet certain USP standards, which isn't the same thing as the product itself meeting USP standards.

Two issues account for almost all of the serious adverse effects concerning herbs: mistaken plant identity and contaminated herbal products. Knowing what you're buying can go a long way toward protecting yourself from these risks.

Always determine whether the herb was "wild-crafted," meaning picked in the wild, or grown as a crop. Sometimes, wild-crafting results in the wrong plants being used in the final product. Small local companies may not have quality-control methods in place that formally identify each batch of collected or purchased herbs. You may decide that it's best to stick with larger companies and standardized products.

It's scary to think that some products on the market contain potentially hazardous contaminants such as toxic plants, heavy metals, or even prescription drugs. Every year, the FDA finds products with dangerous elements like these; the products almost always originate in Asia where government regulations aren't as stringent as they are here. A few herb manufacturers in India and China use traditional practices that many

Western countries consider to be dangerous, such as adding heavy metals or very toxic herbs to their remedies.

Some manufacturers secretly add prescription drugs to traditional remedies to increase the effects of the herbal product—and to increase the company's profits from its sale. Such products, which tend to originate in Hong Kong and Taiwan, are occasionally sold in the United States, too. Not all herbal products from Asian countries are dangerous, but it pays to be cautious. Consult an expert to help you check the plant names on the label; many products from Asia don't use standard botanical names or may misspell them. If you can't clearly identify the plants in the product, don't use it.

It's always best to buy from responsible manufacturers that make their products with appropriate care and attention. They have a vested interest in seeing that consumers get a quality product that works. Not all companies feel this way, and a few just want to make a quick buck—so buyer beware. The American Herbal Products Association (www.ahpa.org) is a trade organization dedicated to the production of high-quality herbs and the development of standards in the manufacture and labeling of herbal products. Membership in the AHPA requires responsible adherence to the association's standards.

For additional information about the quality of herbal products, you can contact the American Botanical Council (ABC), 6200 Manor Road, Austin, Texas 78723. Phone: 512-926-4900. Fax: 512-926-2345. Web site: www.herbalgram.org

A number of magazines publish information about herbal products that is generally reliable. Some of these are listed in appendix B. One notable resource is an educational journal titled *HerbalGram,* which offers an excellent catalog of resources for reliable information about herbal medicine. Published by the American Botanical Council, this journal provides reliable and detailed (if somewhat technical) reports on herbal product safety and efficacy issues. You'll find helpful information about products to avoid, as well as responsible reporting on herb studies. You may also want to check out www.consumerlabs.com for the results of their independent quality tests of herbal products.

❧ ❧ ❧

The safety of any substance you ingest—food, herb, or drug—can never be 100 percent guaranteed. Even if a particular herb has been used safely by others, it may have unexpected or unpleasant side effects for you. You may be allergic to it, as any food, herb, or drug can provoke an allergy. Educating yourself about the plant is the first step; the next step is finding out about safe use. Safety of drugs, herbs, or foods is always relative; some are safer than others.

Fortunately, a thorough search of the medical and herbal literature has turned up only a handful of isolated cases where babies have suffered side effects from herbs their mothers took while nursing. Apparently, there are no recorded cases of a baby suffering serious, lasting harm when his mother ingested herbs. Perhaps this is because nursing mothers are naturally careful about the products they consume. Or it may be due to the fact that so little of any one constituent of an herb actually makes its way into breast milk. Regardless, you should talk to your healthcare provider before taking any herb or herbal product. Please review appendix C for safety ratings of various herbs. Consider this as merely a starting point for the information you should gather.

$\mathscr{Y}$our Healthcare Options

MAKING GOOD CHOICES

You have many choices when it comes to healthcare. Choice is a wonderful thing, but choosing a healthcare provider who meets your needs isn't always easy. How do you choose from the many different healthcare practices and practitioners? And how can you be sure that the provider you choose is actually qualified to help you and your breastfeeding baby?

How do you know which choices are appropriate and effective for nursing mothers (or anyone else, for that matter)? Online you can find all kinds of "magic cures" and just as many "miraculous healers," but how do you know what works and what doesn't? How can you avoid falling prey to a "healer" who claims to be knowledgeable but may do you and your baby more harm than good?

This chapter will help guide you through the sometimes confusing world of healthcare options and healing practices. It introduces you to groups of practitioners and healing systems, with a focus on those remedies and techniques that apply to nursing mothers or their helpers.

Whether you seek medical help from conventional or alternative practitioners, this chapter can help you make decisions about what course of treatment may be best for you as a nursing mother. You'll learn how to look at healthcare practices with an eye to how they impact breastfeeding. Armed with this knowledge, you can more easily find a provider who is truly able to help take care of you and your child.*

Western, or Conventional, Medicine

A majority of Americans view Western medicine as the common or conventional course of action when seeking treatment for an illness. Other forms of medicine may therefore seem unconventional—yet, they are quite conventional to people in other parts of the world who have used them for thousands of years. For the purposes of this book, the term "conventional" is used to refer to Western medicine; the term "unconventional" describes those practices that are, from the Western medical viewpoint, not as usual or as widely accepted. But what is conventional or unconventional to you as a consumer really depends on your own background and beliefs.

Western medicine uses scientific thought as the basis for research and practice. A medical doctor looks at a patient's symptoms and makes a diagnosis based on a scientific definition of the illness and a theory of what might have caused it. The doctor then prescribes a treatment (a drug, surgery, a change in diet) that has been shown to be safe and effective, according to scientific studies of groups of people who have responded to the treatment. Yet, Western medicine isn't only a science—it's also an art. A doctor who is skilled in the art of medicine looks at the patient as an individual and determines which treatment will work based on knowledge of the person's beliefs, concerns, and medical history.

---

* Nonphysical interventions, general massage, exercise programs, and energetic healing systems are not discussed here; neither are healing practices such as biofeedback, Healing Touch, or therapies using color, music, or art. While these practices are valuable for some people and do not present any known risk for breastfeeding, they are beyond the scope of this book.

In his book *Spontaneous Healing,* Dr. Andrew Weil points out how well Western medicine can diagnose and treat people in a crisis (heart attack, trauma sustained in a car accident, or any other situation where someone would be likely to call 911). He makes the point that Western medicine is also helpful for complex medical problems, for conditions that require surgery, and for the prevention of disease through immunization. But Western medicine has its limits. It cannot treat most viral infections, manage some types of mental illness, or cure many degenerative diseases or all cancers.

At times, conventional medicine may be your best healthcare option, especially if the symptoms you have are severe, persistent, or unusual. At other times, you may not want or need the advice of a medical doctor or the use of a prescription drug. What if your situation is fairly simple—for example, you have a cold? While this problem can be bothersome, it doesn't necessarily require a visit to a doctor. In such a situation, there are herbs and other therapies that can help relieve your symptoms.

Today, many people are interested in the healing systems that are widely used in other parts of the world. Patients in the United States are exploring complementary therapies that may help support the conventional treatments recommended by their doctors. Patients are also learning about alternative therapies that can be used instead of drugs or surgery. Western medicine has responded by recognizing the value of other healing systems. These days, you can find doctors who practice a more integrative approach—one that is based on the scientific principles of Western medicine and incorporates not only the patient's own beliefs and customs but also ancient healthcare practices and remedies still new to Western medicine.

Complementary and Alternative Medicine (CAM)

Simply put, alternative therapies are those used *instead of* conventional medicine; complementary therapies are those used *in addition to* conventional medicine. CAM therapies are currently considered unconventional ("not usual and widely accepted") from the standpoint of conventional medicine. Of course, what is considered unconventional today can become commonplace tomorrow.

More and more healthcare providers, including medical doctors, are integrating CAM therapies into Western medicine. This is because many illnesses are better treated with a range of therapies, conventional and unconventional. For example, a patient who has been diagnosed with postpartum depression may benefit from options other than prescription drugs. She and her provider may decide on a program of exercise, counseling, and herbal remedies instead.

One thing that most CAM (or integrative) healthcare practitioners have in common is that they place the individual at the center of care. They are trained to be responsive to the beliefs, words, and actions of the individual seeking help. The practitioner is, ideally, a skilled and informed guide whose aim is to treat the whole human being—mind, body, and spirit. In conventional medicine, the relationship between a doctor and a patient generally isn't viewed as equal; the doctor is the authority, and the patient is expected to merely follow the doctor's advice. Fortunately, doctor-patient relationships are changing for the better in Western medicine, mainly as a result of consumer demand for patients' rights.

For any serious illness, it is recommended that you get a specific diagnosis from a medical doctor before seeking CAM therapies. The doctor will suggest a treatment, but you still have the option of trying alternative or complementary therapies. Once you've looked at all of your choices carefully, it is wise to go back to your doctor and talk about the risks and benefits of the other treatments you're considering. An open-minded and broadly informed physician will take your options seriously and discuss the pros and cons with you.

Sometimes, conventional treatments cause nasty side effects or complications. A complementary treatment may help prevent or lessen such side effects. On the other hand, some complementary treatments may interfere or react badly with conventional ones. There are also risks to foregoing conventional treatments in favor of alternatives, so the risks of any healthcare choice must be carefully weighed. (Foregoing conventional cancer treatments carries great risk, while occasional use of alternative remedies for minor indigestion does not.) For these reasons, it is wise to get a medical diagnosis for a serious or persistent health condition first, and equally important to inform your doctor of any CAM therapies you want to use.

Once you've assembled your health team, keep each member up to date about your medications and therapies. The flow of information will help you benefit from each team member's knowledge and skills.

If you seek help outside of the conventional medical care system, there are some criteria to keep in mind, particularly if you are nursing a baby. The alternative or complementary practitioner you choose should:

- give you individualized attention, analyze your situation from a patient-centered perspective, and suggest treatments that won't interfere with breastfeeding

- allow you to choose among options that don't require you and your baby to be separated

- be informed about breastfeeding and mindful of suggesting treatments that won't cause your breasts pain or discomfort

- avoid recommending megahigh doses of dietary supplements, particularly vitamins or purified isolated substances from medicinal plants (options that aren't as safe for nursing mothers)

- only recommend herbs that are considered safe for a nursing mother

- have experience in assessing the risks or benefits of a treatment for a nursing mother

- be open to working closely with a lactation specialist who can help guide both of you

- ask for your medical history or request that you see a physician to obtain a medical diagnosis first, especially if your situation is complex or serious

- encourage you to keep your doctor informed of what you are doing to address a problem and how the treatment is working for you

- offer to work with your doctor or other healthcare providers

- have the appropriate credentials or experience

Few medical doctors have expertise in alternative and complementary healing; indeed, most have only rudimentary knowledge of these forms of medicine and may not take them seriously. Dr. Andrew Weil is an exception to this rule. In recent years, he has focused his efforts on

A Note about Credentials

Some credentials are gained by experience, such as an apprenticeship in traditional healing; some are gained through standardized training at accredited schools where a standard examination must be passed. For some therapies, healers must undergo both an apprenticeship and an examination to obtain certification or a license. Licenses are recognized and regulated by the state. However, certification may not be state-recognized or regulated; many CAM certifications are issued by a private organizational body that sets its own requirements. Ask about your practitioner's credentials to better understand his or her background and level of training.

changing both medical school curricula and the medical culture itself to better serve patients. As a result, some medical schools across the United States have expanded their training to include alternative healing, and academic health centers across the country are now teaching the principles of integrative medicine. While it is still difficult to find a doctor who is experienced in or knowledgeable about CAM therapies, this situation is beginning to change.

Finding doctors and other healthcare professionals who are informed about breastfeeding can be equally challenging, as this aspect of medical education is still lacking. You may well know more than your doctor does about breastfeeding. If you're a knowledgeable consumer with some basic education in natural medicine or breastfeeding, you are in a good position to evaluate how informed your healthcare professional is.

As a nursing mother, your need for a highly skilled and responsive healthcare provider is doubled because there are two individuals to consider: you and your child. Some practitioners who see lots of mothers and babies may have learned how important it is to protect, support, and promote breastfeeding, but others have not. How can you tell who is supportive and who isn't? And how do you know whether the provider is knowledgeable enough to help you should breastfeeding problems occur?

According to Dr. Jack Newman, who is both a pediatrician and a respected expert on breastfeeding, there are ways to judge your provider's support for and knowledge of breastfeeding. Dr. Newman has shared these ideas in patient handouts and in his famous lectures. Here are Dr. Newman's "red flags" that may indicate a healthcare professional is *not* supportive of breastfeeding:

- He or she gives you formula samples or literature from one or more formula companies when you are pregnant or soon after you have had your baby.

- He or she tells you that a particular brand of formula is best.

- She or he tells you that breastfeeding and bottle-feeding are essentially the same.

- She or he tells you that it is not necessary to breastfeed the baby immediately after birth, since you will be too tired and the baby is often not interested anyway.

- He or she tells you that there is no such thing as nipple confusion and that you should start giving bottles early to your baby to make sure he will accept the bottle nipple.

- She or he tells you that you must stop breastfeeding because you are ill, or your baby is ill, or you need medications or medical tests.

- He or she is surprised to learn that your six-month-old is still breastfeeding.

- He or she tells you that there is no value in breast milk after the baby reaches a certain age—six months, twelve months, whenever.

- He or she tells you that you must never allow your baby to fall asleep at the breast.

- She or he tells you not to stay in the hospital to breastfeed your sick child because it is important for you to rest at home.

Dr. Newman further recommends: "If your medical advisor makes these statements, don't accept them at face value. Ask for more information. Ask for a second opinion—and look for someone with expertise in breastfeeding." You can read Dr. Newman's informative patient handout (handout #18) in its entirety at www.breastfeedingonline.com.

When you visit your healthcare provider, look around for clues as to whether the environment is breastfeeding friendly:

- Do you see pictures of nursing mothers and information about La Leche League meetings? Or are there displays of marketing materials from formula companies (posters, pens, notepads, free samples)?

- Are there are other nursing mothers in the waiting room?

- Does your provider offer information on breastfeeding, contact information for breastfeeding specialists, and schedules for La Leche League meetings?

- Are you given support materials, such as pamphlets and videos about breastfeeding, or are you handed free samples of baby formula?

- Does your provider discuss how to get breastfeeding off to a good start, as well as offer strategies for keeping breastfeeding on track?

- Have you been offered information about reliable books on breastfeeding?

Most importantly, find a provider who listens to you, respects your ideas, understands your needs, and gives you a feeling of trust and confidence. This kind of support is invaluable.

Many nursing mothers have found that expressing how they feel about certain health treatments has encouraged their providers to look for other options and choices. You might say this, for example: "I want to stay on track with breastfeeding, and I feel that the treatment you've recommended isn't compatible with breastfeeding." Or: "Breastfeeding is very important to me and my baby, so I feel that weaning isn't acceptable at this time." Given the opportunity, your provider may discuss alternative therapies or give you the names of others who are better equipped to help you. If you are assertive about what you know and make a point of sharing your feelings about breastfeeding, your provider will probably be happy to listen and respond. If not, it may be time to look elsewhere.

Traditional Healing

Our ancestors knew how to survive and thrive in the wild, and their teachings have come down to us as traditional knowledge of what worked well for untold numbers of generations. Healers taught each generation which plants were to be used for food, medicine, and clothing. Today, however, we are much less connected to the roots of life and are largely insulated from the wild places that human beings once knew well.

Viewed through the tiny window of modern times, traditional wisdom and healing may seem odd, quaint, or possibly unsound. And yet, even within the small time frame of our lives, scientists have reached a new understanding of and appreciation for the healing practices of our ancestors. These healing techniques, after all, weren't invented out of thin air. They are the result of thousands and thousands of years of experience with the living world of plants, animals, and human beings. The science of traditional medicine is based on the collective observations, hands-on experience, and knowledge of generations of healers who left behind their records and teachings.

Three traditional healing systems are discussed here: Traditional Chinese Medicine, Ayurveda, and Western herbal medicine, all of which are ancient, widespread, and extremely influential. Although many other cultures have equally old and valuable models for medicine, they are beyond the scope of this book. For more information about other healing systems, see appendix B.

Traditional Chinese Medicine

Traditional Chinese Medicine, or TCM, is based on the remedies and practices of the indigenous peoples of Asia; its first recorded texts date back nearly 5,000 years. In this ancient system for understanding and treating the human condition, illness is thought of as an imbalance, and treatments are designed to help patients regain their state of balance, or health.

Many of the techniques and remedies used in TCM are fully described in the world's oldest written records. Thousands of years of careful experimentation and recording of results have gone into developing this form of medicine. TCM represents intact knowledge and hands-on skill, passed down from one generation of trained healers to the next. But even though the ancient Chinese characters have been translated into English, the translations are not exact, and the concepts of TCM cannot be perfectly expressed in Western terms.

Practitioners of Traditional Chinese Medicine are adept at assessing all aspects of the patient. They conduct a complete physical exam and ask questions about the patient's diet and daily activities. The diagnosis is a TCM diagnosis—one that doesn't have an equivalent in conventional medicine. The TCM practitioner has a vast and complex array of treatments to choose from and strives to match the treatment(s) to the individual patient's needs. Herbal remedies are selected if the practitioner considers them appropriate. Physical techniques such as acupuncture, acupressure, cupping, and massage may similarly be selected. Or the practitioner may recommend dietary or exercise programs.

Of these therapies, acupuncture, in particular, has gained widespread acceptance within Western conventional medical settings, although it isn't always practiced in a fully traditional manner. Conventional doctors are also investigating herbal remedies within a Western diagnostic framework. But patients who are given Chinese herbal remedies or acupuncture without having had a full TCM evaluation and diagnosis may not be realizing the full benefits of these remedies. Before using ancient herb combinations or other TCM treatments, it is best to have an actual TCM diagnosis from a qualified practitioner.

Traditional Chinese Medicine views the nursing mother and her child as an interconnected and interacting unit. In general, it assumes that what is good for the mother is good for the baby. However, certain TCM remedies and treatments are unsuitable during breastfeeding. As a nursing mother, you need to be sure that the traditional Chinese practitioner you're consulting is truly knowledgeable about Chinese herbal products. Some alternative practitioners have dabbled in Chinese medicine and, on a very slim basis of knowledge, feel confident in directing patients—even nursing mothers—to take Chinese herbal products.

I know of one case in which a nursing mother with chronic sinusitis was advised by her chiropractor to purchase three expensive herbal products made in China. The mother told me that the practitioner selling the products had told her that she'd taken a two-week course on Chinese herbs. The mother was prudent and came to me seeking more information. As it turned out, several of the ingredients in the products were inappropriate for the nursing mother; some of the plants listed on the labels contained aristolochic acid, which is a known kidney toxin. (Plants and herbal products containing aristolochic acid are banned from being imported into the United States.) Treatment with these plants requires careful direction by a skilled TCM practitioner to avoid harming the patient. The lesson here is that an introductory course on Chinese herbal remedies cannot prepare a provider to properly and safely treat patients. It takes years of learning and practice for a TCM practitioner to reach even minimal competency.

To take full advantage of the vast store of wisdom and knowledge that TCM offers, you must choose a skilled, bona fide practitioner. You can look for an Oriental Medicine Doctor (OMD) or a Doctor of Oriental Medicine (DOM); both are trained in the many modalities of Chinese medicine, not just acupuncture. However, DOM is a credential that hasn't been given to practitioners since the early 1980s; current accreditation requires more training.

Look for practitioners who have a master's or doctorate degree from a program approved by the Accreditation Commission for Acupuncture and Oriental Medicine (ACAOM). The National Certification Commission for Acupuncture and Oriental Medicine (NCCAOM) offers certification in three areas of TCM to those who have passed an examination. Most states grant an acupuncture license to those trained through ACAOM programs and certified through the NCCAOM examination. (See appendix B for contact information for these organizations.) Many conventional medical settings offer acupuncture therapy; practitioners should hold a state license such as CA, which stands for Certified in

Acupuncture; LAc and LicAc also indicate a license in acupuncture. Designations such as RAc (Registered Acupuncture) and Dipl Ac (Diploma of Acupuncture) signify at least basic training in acupuncture.

Ayurvedic Medicine

"Ayurveda" describes not only the system of medicine that originated in India but also a way of life. *Ayus* means "life" and *veda* means "knowledge of science," which together can be translated as "science of life." This science seeks to provide wisdom and healing as a way to promote life, health, and happiness.

Ayurveda considers the accumulation of toxicity to be an important explanation for illness. Ayurvedic medicine is based on a system of body types *(doshas)* and employs techniques and remedies to heal the individual based on his or her body type. The Ayurvedic medical writings of India are considered the oldest in the world, predating even those of China, though they aren't as extensive as Chinese medical writings.

The ancient practice of Ayurveda includes the use not only of medicinal plants but also certain animal and mineral products, such as gemstones. The most important herbs used in India (and in China) are slowly being adopted by Western medical herbalists and practitioners. Occasionally, medicinal products imported from India have been found to contain heavy metals such as lead and mercury—not as contaminants but as deliberate ingredients. The importation of such products is illegal in the United States, and good practitioners avoid using them.

In the United States today, finding a practitioner who is fully trained in the traditional Ayurvedic manner can be challenging. According to Dr. Andrew Weil, the Maharishi Mahesh Yogi and his organization provide training and issue certification to physicians as Ayurvedic practitioners "after minimal exposure to the philosophy and methods of the system." Dr. Weil suggests looking for a bona fide traditional practitioner by asking for assistance from the Indian community.

Other experts suggest finding an MD, an osteopath, or a naturopathic physician who has trained in Ayurveda. (Most train in India where schooling extends for several years.) Fully trained practitioners may hold both a Bachelor of Ayurvedic Medicine and Surgery (BAMS) and a Master of Ayurvedic Science (MASc). As yet, Ayurvedic medicine isn't recognized in the United States as a distinct medical system, and no state license or national certification has been developed.

As a nursing mother, you should get to know the views of a prospective practitioner before seeking treatment, because some traditional Ayurvedic practices contradict current recommendations for breastfeeding. For example, in traditional practice, it is customary to give a newborn honey and ghee (a product derived from butter) in the first few days after birth while waiting for the mother's mature milk to come in. Some books on Ayurvedic medicine also state that breastfeeding during certain maternal illnesses and during pregnancy could harm a child.

Because lactation specialists view colostrum, or first milk, as vital to infants, mothers are encouraged to begin breastfeeding as soon as possible after giving birth. Lactation specialists also know that breastfeeding doesn't necessarily have to stop during illness or pregnancy. Before choosing an Ayurvedic practitioner, carefully interview several of them about the therapies they use with nursing mothers. Ask each practitioner about his or her recommendations for fasting, laxatives, and enemas while breastfeeding. (Such treatments are not usually considered appropriate for nursing mothers.) If you're in doubt about a practitioner's views and skills, you should seek a second opinion from another Ayurvedic expert and talk to a lactation specialist.

Western Herbal Medicine

Western herbal medicine is a smorgasbord of herbal traditions and therapies borrowed from and influenced by many peoples in many places, including the healing traditions and herbal remedies of Ancient Greece, Rome, the Middle East, Europe, and the First Nations of the United States, Canada, and Mexico. More recently, the most famous and widely used herbs of China, India, and South America are being incorporated into Western herbalism as well. Herbal medicine continues to grow and change as promising new remedies and approaches become known.

Unlike TCM or Ayurvedic medicine, there is no one system or framework of ideas in Western herbalism. Some medically oriented herbalists use herbs in the same way they use medicines (take "this" herb for "that" symptom); other herbalists use herbs based on different ideas of health and healing. For example, the idea of "humors," which has its roots in both European and Native American medicine, is widely employed by many traditional herbalists. In the humoral view, hot remedies oppose cold conditions and moist herbs are supposed to relieve dryness, so a cool drying herb such as sage would be prescribed to relieve the heat and perspiration of hot flashes. A few Western herbalists may suggest rather strong remedies, such as huge doses of cayenne pepper and stimulant laxatives. These remedies may not be gentle enough for breastfeeding babies and need to be approached with great caution, regardless of how enthusiastic the herbalist may be.

With such a variety of herbs and traditions to draw from, not all practitioners are equally prepared or grounded. Finding a qualified Western herbalist can be a challenge. Self-styled dabblers and those selling the latest herbal "wonder" products have slowed the advancement of traditional herbal medicine. Some blame this problem on the lack of credentialing standards. In the United States, anyone who wishes to call himself or herself an herbalist can do so. However, the American Herbalists Guild (AHG) registry is strict about its Master Herbalist title; only those herbalists who have had years of successful practice and have met other criteria are included on the registry. In fact, some states have only one or two practitioners on the AHG referral list. And in England, the title of Medical Herbalist is earned only after a thorough education in herbalism and modern medical concepts. (See the listings for the American Herbalists Guild and the National Institute of Medical Herbalists in the United Kingdom in appendix B.)

While the American Herbalists Guild is very strict about assigning the title Master Herbalist, it will accept as a general member anyone who wishes to join. Keep in mind that someone who is an AHG member isn't necessarily on the Master Herbalist referral list and may not have the skills you're looking for.

There are many books on Western herbal medicine. Unfortunately, these books often contain out-of-date information about breastfeeding. As you consult these books, you will probably come across general warnings about the use of plants and herbs during breastfeeding, but many herbs are, in fact, quite safe for nursing mothers. Review chapter 4 for an up-to-date discussion of how herbs may affect nursing mothers and their babies.

In addition, many herb books offer traditional information on the practice of treating even very young infants with herbal medicines. What may have been safe for our ancestors doesn't appear to be as risk-free anymore because people today—especially babies—are more prone to food allergies, allergy-related diseases like asthma, and autoimmune diseases. Be aware that these traditional practices may not be appropriate for your infant.

Other CAM Therapy Options

Following are descriptions of other complementary and alternative therapies you may be interested in.

Naturopathy

Naturopathy is based on the idea that good health can best be achieved or maintained by taking advantage of the natural healing powers in all human beings and by using "natural substances" for healing. Most legitimate practitioners receive four years of basic training in biosciences, then complete an additional postgraduate four-year training program at one of two accrediting universities in the United States. A graduate must pass a licensing examination to practice as a Naturopathic Doctor, or ND. Some states recognize and license naturopaths; some don't.

In general, doctors of naturopathy avoid conventional mainstays of treatment, such as drugs or surgery, preferring instead a wide range of "natural" therapies (water massage, acupuncture, or herbal and nutritional therapies, for example). Nutritional therapy can include dietary counseling as well as the use of nutraceuticals, which are products derived from herbs or other natural sources and often formulated in new ways. Be warned that many nutraceutical products are quite costly and should be used with caution when breastfeeding an infant, as they haven't been proven safe by scientific research or traditional knowledge. (Read more about these products in chapter 4.)

On the whole, while naturopaths may be helpful, they may not be particularly knowledgeable about breastfeeding. Some may suggest that you need expensive supplements to make "good" breast milk, but you don't really need them. Other naturopaths may recommend megadoses of vitamins, not realizing that some vitamin and mineral supplements— for example, vitamin A—can enter breast milk in potentially dangerous amounts. Whenever expensive dietary supplements are recommended, be sure to ask the practitioner about alternatives. If you're in doubt about the recommendations, seek out a knowledgeable breastfeeding helper for further information.

Chiropractic and Osteopathy

Chiropractic was invented a century ago by practitioners who believed that all human health problems originated in the spine. Since then, many styles of chiropractic medicine have been developed. A Doctor of Chiropractic (DC) receives four years of undergraduate biosciences training and completes a four-year postgraduate training program approved by the Commission on Accreditation of the Council on Chiropractic Education. Chiropractic doctors are certified by the National Board of Chiropractic Examiners.

Some chiropractors tend to place too much emphasis on the spine and how manipulation of the spine can "cure all." Yet, others can be very helpful in relieving acute musculoskeletal pain, headaches, and chronic pain. Like naturopathic doctors, a chiropractor may suggest herbs, nutraceuticals, vitamins, minerals, and dietary changes. While expertise varies, many chiropractic doctors are well educated in the areas of diet, exercise, and lifestyle counseling.

If you see a chiropractor, be aware that he or she may not be informed about breastfeeding issues (though many of them take a special interest). Some chiropractic doctors may suggest nutraceuticals or herbal medicines without understanding how they may affect a nursing mother or her child. Consider whether the chiropractor you see has any lactation expertise.

Like chiropractors, osteopaths can help both chronic and acute musculoskeletal problems, but they are generally more competent than chiropractors due to their more extensive training. A Doctor of Osteopathy (DO) receives much of the same training as a conventional medical doctor: four years of undergraduate work in bioscience, another four years of study at an osteopathic medical school, a one-year internship, and another two to six years in a residency program. Osteopathic doctors are board certified by the National Board of Osteopathic Medical Examiners and are licensed to practice medicine in all fifty states.

Osteopathic manipulative therapy, or OMT, is designed to help relieve pain and illness. One form of OMT is cranial therapy, which can be particularly helpful for ear infections. Cranial therapy has also helped some infants who have difficulty breastfeeding. Before considering OMT, discuss the treatment with your lactation specialist; and be sure to select an osteopath who has experience working with breastfeeding infants.

Aromatherapy

Aromatherapy, a term coined in the 1920s, simply means the use of essential oils as therapeutic agents. (See chapter 4 for more on essential oils.) An essential oil is the ultimate concentrate of a plant's aroma—for example, the perfume of a flower or the scent of a crushed leaf or root. These preparations are highly concentrated and highly potent; typically, they are used in very small amounts after dilution in other oils or water. Essential oils have an aroma that is thought to affect the emotions as well as the body; depending on the type of oil and how it is diluted, you can add it to bathwater, inhale the vapors, or apply it to your skin. While these oils may lift your mood or calm you down, they are also intended to assist in healing. If you have a head cold, for example, you may be relieved by a steamy bath filled with just the right amount of peppermint and thyme oil, which can clear your sinuses and comfort your soul. Also, thyme's essential oil (like that of many other plants) is antimicrobial and anti-inflammatory; inhaling its components can help your body fight off the virus that is causing your head cold.

When you are breastfeeding a baby, you must use essential oils with care. Knowledgeable aromatherapists should be able to tell you how to use essential oils safely, but an alarming number of books on the topic don't include adequate warnings. Be sure to determine first whether the oil you want to use is potentially toxic, irritant, or allergenic. Only use oils that are gentle and unlikely to cause a problem for you or your baby. Avoid using essential oils on or near the breast; because they're oily, they leave a residue on the skin that a breastfeeding baby is likely to ingest. A few essential oils can cause breathing problems when used near a baby's face. (See chapter 10 for information on using essential oils in your baby's bath and on your baby's skin.) Question any aromatherapist who proposes applying essential oils to your breasts and chest. In general, such products will need to be washed off before breastfeeding.

Homeopathy

Traditional herbal medicine (as practiced in most of the world), the use of nutraceuticals, and Western medicine all share one thing in common: they are essentially allopathic. Allopathic remedies attempt to correct a problem through opposition. In other words, they act against something in the body that is causing illness or blocking the recovery of health. For example, antibiotics (note the prefix *anti-*) work against bacteria by killing them off and restoring the body to health. Similarly, antiemetics stop vomiting by countering the development of nausea in the body.

Homeopathy, on the other hand, is a two-hundred-year-old system of diagnosis and treatment guided by the idea that "like treats like." In this health system, the patient's list of symptoms is carefully described; a remedy that produces the same symptoms in overdose is then offered in an extremely diluted (and thus safe) amount.

Homeopathic remedies and publications on homeopathy are widely available in health-food stores. A particularly helpful source of information on the topic is *Homeopathy Today,* a journal published by the National Center for Homeopathy. It can usually be found in health-food stores.

Many mild illnesses (such as colds) can be self-treated with home-opathics. But if you have a more complex or chronic condition, it is best to see a homeopathic practitioner first, instead of purchasing and using a remedy on your own. Currently, homeopaths get their training and practice from a wide variety of schools. Homeopaths can be certified in their field as a Certified Classical Homeopath, or CCH. Look for this credential if you're trying to find a skilled practitioner. In the United States, few medical doctors are also homeopaths; in Europe, however, there are homeopathic medical clinics and even hospitals.

Bodywork and Massage Therapies

There are a bewildering number of types of bodywork, massage, and other touch-based therapies. In the United States, the training and credentials of the massage therapist (MT) varies from state to state. An MT may have received training from a program approved by the Commission on Massage Therapy Accreditation, or he or she may be certified by the National Certification Board for Therapeutic Massage and Bodywork and hold a license to practice.

Many massage therapists have received training in a variety of breast massage techniques that were developed in Asia (particularly Japan). Be aware that some of these techniques aren't advisable for nursing mothers, as they may cause pain. Breast massage should never hurt; do not allow a massage therapist to cause pain or discomfort to your breasts. You can read more about breast massage in chapter 8.

🌿 🌿 🌿

You know yourself better than anyone. As a nursing mother in close contact with your baby, you also know your baby best. When it comes to matters of health, do not be afraid to speak in a strong voice. Share your thoughts with your healthcare provider; ask for information and resources when you need help. If you aren't satisfied, ask more questions. Keep an open mind so that you hear what your provider is saying, but always know that you have the option to seek other treatments if you want. When all is said and done, you know best what will or won't work in your situation. Your healthcare provider may be your guide, but you are the one in the driver's seat.

$\mathcal{P}$ostpartum Recovery

TAKING CARE OF YOURSELF AFTER DELIVERY

Although much has been written about herbs and postpartum recovery, the current literature rarely includes information about herbs that are safe and beneficial for nursing mothers. This chapter offers up-to-date information on herbs and other comfort measures that can help you heal after childbirth. Each aspect of your postpartum recovery can impact breastfeeding; the more quickly you recover, the more quickly you can get up to speed with nursing your baby. Because another important aspect of recovery is taking good care of yourself, you'll also find suggestions for how to eat well, prevent fatigue, and maintain your health during this exciting, but exhausting, time of life.

What to Expect after Delivery

After you have given birth, your uterus will contract into what feels like a hard ball. You can feel your uterus by pressing into your abdomen below the bellybutton; it should feel solid and firm. Over the next ten days, it will shrink in size to the point where you will no longer be able to locate it by feeling your abdomen. After about five to six weeks, your uterus will return to near its pre-pregnant size.

You will most likely have cramping sensations that indicate uterine contractions. The hormone oxytocin plays a role in these contractions. As your baby breastfeeds, he stimulates your nipples, releasing oxytocin, which not only contracts your uterus but causes milk to flow from your breasts. Frequent breastfeeding after birth will help your uterus to shrink—and allow you to get your figure back faster.

Postpartum uterine cramps are normal, and they will be stronger with each baby. (The cramps are known as after-pains.) Women having their second and third babies find the after-pains as intense as labor pains. After-pains are worsened whenever the uterus relaxes a bit, allowing blood to pool before suddenly contracting again. Because breastfeeding stimulates a smooth and sustained uterine contraction, the after-pains pass more quickly if you breastfeed (although they may be more intense during breastfeeding). The worst of the after-pains are usually over in about two days. Applying warm, moist packs over the area can help ease the discomfort. You can also use anti-inflammatory pain medications such as ibuprofen.

Certain herbs can help relieve uterine cramping while stimulating a smooth and sustained contraction. (Such herbs can similarly work to relieve menstrual cramping.) To ease after-pains, herbalist Susun Weed suggests sipping a black haw or cramp bark tea throughout the day, drinking one to two cups of ground ivy tea per day, or drinking catnip leaf tea "freely." (The catnip tea is quite delicious.) She notes that repeated use of catnip tincture can lead to significant sedation, so nursing mothers may prefer the tea instead. Another suggested remedy is taking five to twenty drops of motherwort tincture, using the smallest dose that works. See chapter 4 for information about tinctures.

If simple comfort remedies like these don't seem to relieve your cramps, talk to your doctor. Severe cramping may occur with serious bleeding or may indicate other complications. (See "The Danger of Hemorrhage" on the following page.)

The Danger of Hemorrhage

Postpartum hemorrhage (loss of more than two cups of blood) can occur when the uterus relaxes and loses tone. If at any time in the first few hours or days after giving birth you experience a heavy flow and your uterus feels soft or flabby, you can massage it with gentle pressure and circular strokes. Putting your baby to your breast immediately can help your uterus to contract as well.

Herbal preparations, such as red raspberry and nettle tea (with their mild astringent properties) or motherwort tincture, can help prevent postpartum hemorrhage. If hemorrhage does occur, a tincture of shepherd's purse may help. However, you must get medical assistance if you have heavy vaginal bleeding. Call 911 if you have heavy bleeding or are repeatedly passing large clots. If you are experiencing dizziness, nausea, faintness upon sitting or standing, pallor, weakness, restlessness, or thirst, you may be in imminent danger of going into shock. Take the teas or tinctures, but call 911 first.

Sometimes, a slow hemorrhage occurs over many hours or days. Because it doesn't look like a gush of blood, you may assume it's nothing serious. However, symptoms of shock may develop with a slow hemorrhage. Call 911 if you are experiencing any of the symptoms described above.

After your baby is born, your uterus will produce a liquid discharge known as lochia. This flow occurs as the uterine lining returns to its prepregnant state. Here is what you can expect:

- In the first three days: You will have a flow of red blood with mucus and small tissue bits (lochia rubra). The flow should not contain large clots (larger than a quarter) or membranes and should not be excessive. First-time mothers have lesser amounts of lochia. Getting out of bed and moving around increases the flow somewhat, especially after the birth of your first baby. Too much activity too soon will increase the flow of lochia, even after it has slowed and darkened.

- After three days: As the flow continues, the discharge becomes pinker and then yellowish (lochia serosa).

- After ten days: By this point, the discharge should be of a thin or runny consistency; the color is white or almost colorless (lochia alba). The white lochia continues until around six weeks postpartum; when it ceases, the uterus has returned to its normal state.

Use sanitary pads—never tampons—to absorb the lochia. Keep track of how often you change your sanitary pads so that you can gauge whether your flow is normal. Typically, the flow will be as heavy as, or heavier than, a menstrual period for the first three days after childbirth. Your lochia flow will likely be heaviest in the first day after delivery. Having a record of how many pads you are using, and monitoring changes in the color of the flow as well, can be helpful should a problem occur. A note of caution: Bright red blood flow after four days, or a sudden recurrence of bright red flow after the discharge has become dark or pink, is not normal. The lochia should not smell offensive at any time, either.

If you have a heavy lochia flow, repeated large clots, or a persistent or recurring red lochia, you may have fragments of the placenta left in your uterus. Call your doctor immediately to find out whether retained placental fragments might be the cause of your symptoms.

Retained placenta or placental fragments can prevent milk production after birth. If your milk has not come in by the fourth day after your baby's birth and your lochia flow isn't following a normal course, seek a medical evaluation. If the fragments are removed soon enough after birth, there will be a dramatic increase in milk production; however, not all obstetricians understand the importance of looking for fragments right away. If your milk doesn't come in when it's supposed to, the possibility of retained fragments must be investigated, even in the absence of an unusually heavy lochia flow. It takes only a very small fragment of placenta to make enough of the hormone progesterone to block milk production. Some placental conditions—for example, placental accretia—complicate the removal of all of the fragments from the uterus. Ask your doctor if the placenta was normal or not.

You may experience a low-grade fever of up to 100°F in the first day or so after birth, but this type of fever isn't abnormal and isn't likely to last more than twenty-four hours. Even if you have a slight fever, there is no need to stop breastfeeding.

If your fever is accompanied by pain, swelling at your incision sites, foul-smelling lochia, or difficulty with urination, or if you have a fever over 102°F, call your doctor right away. You may have an infection. Urinary tract infections are common after birth. Uterine infections aren't as common, but they are serious and require immediate medical attention.

If you are diagnosed with a uterine infection, do not try to treat yourself. Using an herbal treatment in this case isn't a good idea, because if it doesn't work you risk not only your fertility but also your life. You may use a well-chosen healing herb with a prescribed antibiotic, but not as a substitute for the antibiotic. Almost all antibiotics can be taken while breastfeeding. Talk to a knowledgeable herbalist about healing herbs, and be sure to mention the antibiotics you're taking.

For urinary tract infections, you may want to try yarrow or uva-ursi, which herbalists traditionally describe as "drying" herbs. However, be aware that these two herbs have been known to reduce milk supply in some women when taken internally. Consult a knowledgeable herbalist for more information if you decide to use herbs to fight a urinary tract infection.

If you are prone to repeated urinary infections, drinking cranberry juice can clear up a lingering infection and help prevent recurrences.

(Cranberries contain a substance that interferes with bacteria's ability to cling to the bladder and urethra.) Drink 4–6 oz. of pure cranberry juice or 8 oz. of a cranberry juice blend daily.

If your doctor recommends that you stop nursing while being treated for an infection, know that infections in the mother can usually be treated without disrupting the critical first days of breastfeeding. Babies are not at risk from most maternal bacterial infections; in fact, babies who don't breastfeed are more vulnerable to infection. If your healthcare provider suggests that you should stop breastfeeding altogether or wait until you feel better, it may be time to speak with a lactation specialist or get a second opinion from a different doctor. In almost all cases, breastfeeding can continue during a maternal illness.

Sweating a Lot Is Normal

After birth, many mothers experience drenching perspiration, part of the body's increased elimination of waste products during postpartum recovery. Sweat contains many antibacterial compounds, so all the extra sweating is helpful (if not very pleasant). In the early weeks of breastfeeding, you may experience what feels like a hot flash accompanied by drenching sweat every time you nurse. The heat and sweating come on rapidly with the let-down of your milk. Like menopausal hot flashes, these seem to happen more frequently at night. They will fade with time; until then, drink to quench your thirst, wear layers, and change your bra and shirt frequently, as needed.

Sore Bottom, Tearing, and Stitches

If you have had a vaginal birth, you will probably have some soreness after delivery. Frequent rinsing of the perineum during the early days can soothe some of the pain and will help prevent infections of the urinary tract or vagina. If you had any tearing or an episiotomy, it's important to keep these wounds very clean. You may be given a periwash bottle at the hospital; if not, any kind of clean squirt bottle will do. Gently squirt warm water on the perineum, spraying the water from front to back. Avoid touching the area with your fingers. Always rinse after urinating and especially after having a bowel movement.

Once your stitches or tears have begun to heal, you can add herbal teas to your periwash bottle if you wish. As a precaution, avoid using comfrey tea on open wounds unless you have found a toxin-free product. (See appendix C for more details about comfrey.)

In her book *Herbal Healing for Women*, Master Herbalist Rosemary Gladstar suggests adding some aloe vera gel to the periwash bottle to reduce stinging around the stitches. Every couple of days, make a fresh batch by scraping the gel from a freshly cut aloe vera leaf and adding it to water. Keep this mixture in the refrigerator so it stays cool; use it to replenish your periwash bottle, as needed.

To add to your discomfort, you may suffer a bit of constipation in the early days after birth. If you had hemorrhoids during your pregnancy, they may continue to cause discomfort after birth, or hemorrhoids may occur for the first time. Because it is painful to bear down, hemorrhoids contribute to constipation. Also, the rectum has been stretched during vaginal birth, and perhaps accidentally cut during episiotomy. Rarely, a tear may extend into the rectal muscle; ask your obstetrician what kinds of tears, if any, occurred during birth if you're not sure. For quick pain relief and to reduce swelling from tears and hemorrhoids, use witch hazel on gauze pads or a commercial preparation (like Tucks). You can place the soothing pads directly on your sanitary napkin. Sitz baths with astringent herbs can also help. (See "Sitz Baths" on the following page.)

To relieve constipation, remember the basics: exercise, fiber, and lots of fluids. Get out and walk your baby, if possible. Eat lots of roughage (fruits, vegetables, whole grains). Drink plenty of water and other fluids to help soften the stool. If needed, you can use an over-the-counter stool softener, but choose a mild one to avoid cramping.

Avoid stimulant laxatives or large doses of stimulant herbs. If you decide to use stimulant herbs, always use the smallest dose that works for the shortest period of time. Cascara is the mildest stimulant laxative, but because it is expensive, standardized preparations with well-controlled doses are hard to find. Senna leaf or fruit is another fairly mild laxative. Cheap to produce, it is available in many over-the-counter preparations. (Be careful with the dose you take when your baby is small.) OTC preparations such as Senakot have the advantage of a guaranteed controlled dose, but consult your doctor first. Strong purgatives such as aloe or rhubarb root should be avoided entirely; most herbal products that contain these herbs are inappropriate for nursing mothers, as the dose of active ingredients isn't controlled. Careful reading of products labels that claim to improve bowel function or promote "cleansing" may reveal the presence of such herbs.

Often, mothers start taking iron supplements if they have suffered significant blood loss during birth. If you use iron, be prepared for the constipating effects. To decrease the risk of constipation, add fiber to your diet when taking iron supplements. Alternatively, herbal iron tonics may be less constipating.

Sitz Baths

Sitz baths are a form of hydrotherapy; they are designed to stimulate circulation in the pelvic region, bringing comfort and healing to tissues inside and out. Sitz baths may also offer hemorrhoid relief, especially if astringent herbs are used. If you have stitches, your doctor may recommend a limit of one sitz bath per day at first.

For a hot sitz bath, try the following:

1. Rinse the perineum well so it is clean.

2. Find a container that you can soak your bottom in. Because you'll sit in it for about fifteen minutes, make sure it is big enough that

you won't get stuck. Place the container in the bathtub. A sitz bath pan can be purchased, or one may be given to you in the hospital; the pan is designed to sit on the toilet (both lids up). If you're using a sitz bath pan, rest your feet on a stool or a big book to reduce pressure.

3. Fill the container with water that is comfortably hot, but not burning hot.

4. If desired, you can add herbal infusions to the water; these can be very soothing and may help speed healing. Good herb choices include yarrow, rosemary, goldenseal, oak bark, witch hazel, and myrrh. Just make sure to strain out the herbs first.

5. Soak for fifteen minutes. If the water cools off quickly, you can keep adding more hot water. Don't sit for more than twenty minutes, as nice as the bath may feel.

6. If at any time you start to feel faint or woozy, stop the sitz bath and stand up slowly, hanging onto something. If someone else is nearby, ask this person to help you get to your feet. (It is possible to faint from a hot sitz bath, so it's a good idea to have someone close by, at least the first couple of times.)

A contrast sitz bath uses hot and cold water to vigorously stimulate blood flow. The feeling could be compared to going from a hot sauna into the snow—tingly. To speed the healing of tears and stitches, Rosemary Gladstar suggests taking contrast sitz baths several times a day for at least five days after birth; read her book *Herbal Healing for Women* for a wonderful description of this therapy.

Basically, you need two pans of water for a contrast sitz bath: one as hot as you can stand, the other icy cold. Herbs can be added to the pan of hot water if you wish. Alternately soak in each pan, relaxing in the hot one for a few minutes and then steeling yourself for a dip in the cold one. Try to stay in the cold water for a few minutes, then repeat the entire process at least five times. (A contrast sitz bath can also relieve engorged breasts, using the same basic contrast sitz method; see chapter 8 for more about engorgement.)

Getting Active and Preventing Fatigue

As soon as possible after birth, and when you feel up to it, get out of bed and start walking around. A bit of exercise right away not only makes you feel better but also helps prevent constipation and keeps the uterus toned. The first time out of bed you may experience a gush of lochia, but it should quickly diminish.

If you had a cesarean birth, the postpartum nurses will assist you in getting out of bed. It is recommended that you take the pain medications you're offered so you can begin walking around. Mild activity reduces gas in the belly by stimulating the bowels to start working again. Becoming more active also reduces pain—and, therefore, the need for pain medications—after surgery. Most importantly, getting out of bed and walking as soon as possible reduces the chance of developing a blood clot in the leg and lung. If you start to experience warmth or painful areas in your legs, call your doctor immediately, as you may have developed a blood clot. A clot can be life-threatening and shouldn't be ignored. If you're hospitalized for a blood clot, be assured that there is no medical reason to stop or interrupt breastfeeding. If needed, seek the support of a lactation specialist or La Leche League Leader.

During the postpartum period, pay special attention to your posture and motions throughout the day, whether you're walking the baby or going about your normal tasks. For the first six weeks after the birth of your baby, your pelvic support structures and abdominal muscles may be somewhat weakened, having been stretched out during pregnancy and birth. In addition, the hormones of pregnancy make these support structures more flexible, leaving them more prone to injury after birth. (If you were on bedrest before birth, it will take longer for you to regain your normal strength and muscle tone. Give yourself extra time to recover.) The muscles and supportive structures of your pelvis and back will eventually return to their previous condition, but, meanwhile, use good body mechanics so you don't put undue pressure on your back and hips. Avoid bending over too far and too often, for example. If possible, limit the amount of time you spend carrying your baby around in a car seat–style infant carrier. This type of seat is bulky and awkward to carry, putting stress on your neck and back. Cloth baby carriers (the ones that are supported by shoulder straps and hold the baby against your chest) are a nice option, but they may stress your shoulders once your baby starts to gain weight. Consider purchasing a newborn sling, which will allow you to wrap up your baby and hold him close to you while leaving your arms free. Slings also distribute and balance the weight between your shoulders and hips.

Checking your posture when breastfeeding is important, too. Poor posture can result in pain in your back, neck, arms, wrists, and even in your breasts. If you feel physically uncomfortable while breastfeeding, take a look at your overall posture. Maybe you're hunched over as you feed your baby? Instead, hold your back upright and bring your baby toward you. Check to see that your arms are supported as they hold your baby; if not, they will start to ache. Are you lifting your shoulders? Consciously tell yourself to relax them after your baby is latched. When sitting in a chair, put your feet up on something; nursing stools are ideal, but a coffee table will do.

When you first start breastfeeding, spend time practicing the various holds or positions. You can place a pillow under your arm to help you position your baby near your breast more easily. If necessary, use a second pillow underneath your baby for added support. In appendix A, you'll find a list of books about breastfeeding, many of which include useful tips on posture and positioning.

It probably comes as no surprise to you that life will be especially challenging in the early weeks after birth. Fortunately, this is usually the time when family and friends are eager to be around the new baby and to support you however they can. Feel free to take them up on their offers to help. Let your supporters relieve you of some household tasks—laundry, dishes, clutter, and meals, for example. When you give yourself permission not to worry about these chores, you'll feel a sense of relief. You can then focus on more important things, like breastfeeding and getting the rest you need. Many nursing mothers have realized that the more time they have to focus on breastfeeding in the early days, the more smoothly things go. These mothers are generally less fatigued and better able to heal.

In many places around the world, a mother enjoys about six weeks of solicitous support after delivery; her every need is met by the wise women around her who look after her home, feed her special foods, and offer healing remedies to help her recover physically. This is also a time of teaching and learning. The new mother is shown how to breastfeed and care for her new baby. And wouldn't you know it: women who are supported in these ways rarely experience postpartum depression.

Friends and family will play a critical role in helping you and your baby to get through the early days and weeks. Your first priority is taking care of your baby and yourself. You need time to bond with your child and get breastfeeding off to a good start. Other family members can pitch in by taking over the household tasks and making sure you get healthy meals. It helps to have someone nearby who is willing to hold and snuggle the baby at a moment's notice, so you can take a sitz bath, rest, or sit down for a meal. For many families, the new father plays a vital role in postpartum recovery and breastfeeding support. Be sure to recognize this and encourage him to find breastfeeding-friendly ways to help you and your baby.

Sometimes, new mothers who want to breastfeed exclusively run into resistance from family members or other important people in their lives. For example, other children in the family need attention and may feel left out. Or the baby's father may lament that he doesn't get the opportunity to feed the baby; so might the baby's grandmothers or aunts. In our bottle-feeding culture, people often have a cherished expectation of someday feeding the special new baby in their lives. They may be surprised or hurt if his mother says no.

The experience of countless mothers and their breastfeeding helpers has clearly shown that introducing a bottle in the early weeks can throw breastfeeding off track. Let people know, kindly but firmly, why you are breastfeeding exclusively. Go out of your way to "share" the baby with others when you aren't feeding him—they can change him, bathe him, or simply hold him close. They can even take him on walks to show him off to the world.

Another big payoff of having helpers around you is that they can let you get some sleep. Fatigue is a major challenge for every new mother—and for fathers, too. Breastfeeding around the clock may feel overwhelming at first; it's normal to get tired and fatigued with a newborn in the house.

You may feel that bottle-feeding mothers are getting more sleep than you are, but it's not always true. All newborns need fairly constant attention, no matter how they're fed, and all of them wake at night (usually when you least want them to). At times, you may be tempted to quit breastfeeding, give the baby a bottle, or even let him cry it out. Hold on somehow and focus on finding support. Can someone come over to help with the chores? Ideally, this person can handle the cleaning or other household tasks so you can focus on the more immediate concerns of sleeping, eating, and feeding the baby. Can someone take care of your other children for part of the day or evening, or perhaps carry and comfort your baby in between feedings? This way, you can get a nap or a few hours of uninterrupted sleep, which will feel like a blessing.

When you're tired and fatigued, it's never a good time to make decisions about breastfeeding. Make very sure that you get some rest, some food, and whatever else you need to regain a sense of balance. A nap of one to two hours can do wonders; find a way to take one. Once you've had some sleep, things will look brighter and you can once again find energy to meet your baby's needs.

Eating Well for You and Your Baby

What to feed your baby is simple: breast milk and more breast milk. This will cover his nutritional needs for many months. But what about you? Do you need a degree in nutrition to be assured of making good milk?

Not at all. You don't need a perfect diet to make quality milk in sufficient amounts; your body does that work on its own. However, what you eat is important because a good diet is one of the keys to good health.

Here are some basic tips on eating well:

- Eat a wide variety of foods in as close to their natural state as possible—raw vegetables, fresh fruits, and whole grains. Raw or simply prepared whole foods give you energy and provide an excellent foundation for continued heath.

- A diet that includes lots of different fruits and vegetables provides necessary minerals, vitamins, protein, and fiber. And, as scientific research is proving, fruits and vegetables also offer thousands of naturally occurring plant chemicals that are essential for good health. To get your share of all these wonderful substances (discovered and undiscovered), eat a wide variety of plants, especially brightly colored fruits and vegetables and lots of dark, leafy greens. It is widely recommended that you eat at least five servings of fruits and vegetables per day to optimize your health; this will also optimize your energy.

- To get more nutrients, eat your fruits and vegetables when they're fresh. Whenever possible, eat them raw or lightly cooked. Frozen or canned fruits and vegetables usually don't have as many nutrients as fresh ones, but they are good options if they help you add more plant foods to your overall diet.

- If they're available and affordable, buy good quality organic foods. They have a higher nutritional value and often taste better. Whatever your budget affords, know that eating plenty of fruits and vegetables every day, organic or not, is the important thing.

- Know the value of diversity and variety. Eating smaller amounts of lots of different foods (1) ensures that all your nutritional bases are covered, (2) reduces your breastfeeding baby's risk of developing allergies and food sensitivities, and (3) lessens the likelihood of any unpredictable or undesirable effects from eating excessive amounts of any one thing.

- Stay hydrated by drinking plenty of water, but avoid drinking it to excess. Simply drink enough to quench your thirst. Ironically, drinking much more water than is needed to quench thirst has been found to reduce milk production.

- Drink beverages such as coffee, caffeinated tea, and herbal tea in moderation. These beverages contain plant constituents that, in large amounts, have medicinal properties that may affect your milk supply or, if they contain caffeine, may upset your baby. Varying the herbal teas you consume may help you avoid unwanted medicinal effects.

To learn more about eating healthy, see appendix A for recommended books on breastfeeding, nutrition, and parenting; many of the topics in this chapter are discussed in greater detail in other books for mothers.

News about Fats and Choline

To some extent, what you consume affects the fats and fatty acids in your breast milk, which is one reason to pay attention to the types and amounts of fats you consume. Breast milk normally contains some especially nutritious fats, such as essential omega-3 fatty acids. Breast milk also contains cholesterol, which is important for your baby's development. But if you consume a lot of the saturated fats known as trans-fats, these, too, will enter your milk.

Trans-fats are solid at room temperature and have an artificially altered chemical structure. They are believed to encourage the development of inflammatory processes in the body. In recent years, trans-fats have been linked to obesity, heart disease, and even cancer.

Animal fats, when heated, naturally generate some trans-fats. However, most trans-fats in the American diet come from processed foods. Manufacturers invented "partially hydrogenated" fats as a cheap source of solid fat for making processed food products such as shortening and margarine. These artificially made products are very high in trans-fats.

Besides shortening and margarine, products that contain trans-fats include most deep-fried foods; processed luncheon meats; cookies, pastries, and other bakery goods; most crackers; many brands of chips and other snack foods; and many brands of peanut butter. During the breast-feeding years and beyond, try to minimize your intake of partially hydrogenated fats. You can begin by reading product labels carefully so you know what you're buying. You can also try cooking with less oil, switching to natural peanut butter, and avoiding fast foods as much as possible.

In addition to limiting trans-fats, you should make a point of eating "good" fats like the omega-3s. This is a family of essential fatty acids found in such foods as fish, egg yolks, dark green leafy vegetables, and certain nuts and seeds. They are called essential fatty acids because they are necessary for healthy functioning. The omega-3s are polyunsaturated, like canola, soy, or corn oil, but they have a different structure and are used differently by the body. The body turns one type of omega-3, called alpha-linolenic acid (ALA), into larger and more complex fatty acids, called eicosapentaenoic acid (EPA) and docosahexaenoic acid (DHA). These acids in turn are used by the body to make certain types of prostaglandins—hormonelike substances that specialize in damping down inflammation in the body. Therefore, omega-3s can play an important role in the prevention or improvement of such inflammatory conditions as allergy, arthritis, and cardiovascular disease. They also can play significant roles in maintaining healthy nerve, brain, and retinal tissues. Breast milk naturally contains DHA, which benefits the development of the baby's brain and vision; the higher IQ of breastfed babies is likely due, in part, to the DHA secreted in the milk.

The modern American diet is poor in omega-3s, compared to what people ate just a couple of generations ago. However, it's not difficult to add omega-3s to your diet. Simply eating green foods daily and consuming fish weekly will give you a great start. Leafy greens such as kale, collards, and bok choy, as well as walnuts, pumpkin seeds, and especially flaxseed, are all good sources of ALA. Eating fish, even just 3 oz. once a week, has been shown to have measurable health benefits. Fatty cold-water fish, such as salmon, herring, and codfish, are considered the best sources of omega-3s, but any kind of fish, including tuna, has been shown to have health benefits. Expensive dietary supplements made from algae aren't necessary, but they may be helpful if you don't eat fish products.

Your breast milk naturally contains DHA and ALA, and studies have shown that mothers with low-DHA diets still produce good amounts of DHA in their breast milk—enough to ensure the superior eye and brain development of their babies. Even so, it seems reasonable to take care of your own health by eating generous amounts of healthy foods, including green vegetables and fish. If you hate eating fish, try fish oil capsules. Some people who use fish oil capsules notice that they get "fish burps." If this happens to you, you can try emulsified fish oils. (The orange flavor tastes great.)

Choline is another important part of a healthy diet. This nutrient is abundant in dairy products, meat, egg yolks, and fish. Whole grain rice, barley, oats, wheat, soybeans, and peas are also good sources of choline. In foods, choline is often found as part of a waxy-oily complex called lecithin. Egg yolks and soybeans are particularly rich in lecithin. Soy lecithin is used as an emulsifier in many foods; for example, chocolate is made smooth with lecithin. Lecithin is also available as a nutritional supplement (usually as soy lecithin). You can find it in health-food stores in the form of granules, liquids, and capsules.

Choline is an essential component of cell membranes and is intimately involved in antioxidant activities in the body, helping to reduce homocysteine levels. Homocysteine is an amino acid that has recently been implicated in the development of heart disease and other chronic diseases. Choline plays an important role in fat and cholesterol metabolism and in the transport of fatty substances around the body. This nutrient is needed for normal nervous system activity as well.

Choline is an important constituent of breast milk. Studies of dairy animals have shown that milk production draws on the mother's choline stores in the liver as part of the manufacture and transport of fatty substances used in making milk. It is known that mothers who have repeated plugged milk ducts can often solve the problem by supplementing their diet with a choline source such as soy lecithin. Mothers also find that eating whole grains such as oats daily can help a flagging milk supply. In Japan, nursing mothers often eat whole grain rice to help with an oversupply of milk. (Chapters 7 and 8 discuss breast and milk supply problems.) In short, choline appears to be helpful for many different breastfeeding problems, and while the role this nutrient plays in breastfeeding isn't fully known, it is likely an important one.

It has long been thought that choline requirements for the body are easily met through the typical American diet, but this isn't always the case. Many people currently avoid consuming meat, dairy, and eggs. Yet, these foods are all good sources of lecithin, with egg yolk being the very best. Further, our typical diet base of refined grains actually contains very little choline. You can ensure plentiful choline in your diet by simply eating more eggs per week and adding more whole grains. But if you avoid consuming any animal products, you may need to make a point of eating lots more whole grain rice, barley, oats, or soy products that contain lecithin.

Eating well helps your postpartum recovery and provides a source of energy in the early weeks and months of your baby's life. And what you're eating now sets the stage for your child's diet in the future. In just a few months, he will start on solid foods; soon he will be eating what you eat. Learn to prepare a wide variety of fresh foods so you continue to give him the best in the years to come.

Food Sensitivities and Allergies

Babies cannot be allergic to mother's milk because human protein is nonallergenic. However, nursing mothers should avoid eating large amounts of any one food because this might trigger hypersensitivity or even allergy in their babies. It is known that small amounts of the allergenic constituents of food (usually proteins) can be absorbed into the mother's bloodstream from the gastrointestinal tract and make their way into breast milk.

When large amounts of an allergenic food are eaten, enough of the constituent can enter breast milk to cause a reaction in a very sensitive baby. Before six months of age, babies have "leaky" gastrointestinal tracts, so allergens easily pass into the bloodstream, where they can then cause allergic symptoms. Children who have a food sensitivity may react with some or all of these symptoms: colic, fussiness, thrashing in their sleep, repeated ear infections or frequent colds, eczema, diarrhea, or even blood in the stool. Cow's milk protein is the most common culprit when a baby is showing such symptoms. Other common foods that can trigger reactions are oranges and other citrus fruits, nuts (particularly peanuts), wheat, corn, and sometimes beans and other legumes.

If your baby has a food sensitivity or an allergy, it may still be possible for you to eat a bit of the food that is causing the problem; but larger portions may cause your baby to react. Some mothers find that they must eliminate the problem food for up to three weeks to find out whether it is indeed an allergen. It can sometimes take this long to clearly see an allergy develop, and it may take an equally long time to clear the milk of an allergen. In more severe cases, an onset of allergy is more rapid and clears up just as rapidly when the mother's diet changes.

By eating a diverse diet, you not only offer your baby a variety of nutrients in your milk, but also protect him from developing a potential sensitivity to particular foods. Plus, the milk tastes different every day, which is more interesting to your baby. If at all possible, breastfeed your baby exclusively until he is ready for solid foods; this protects him from consuming large doses of potentially allergenic substances and greatly lessens the risk of developing food allergies once he starts to eat table food.

Another benefit of exclusive breastfeeding is that it is easier to figure out if your baby is reacting to some of the foods you eat. Identifying a food sensitivity is more difficult after your baby is introduced to the wide world of solid foods. If you think your baby is reacting to

Caffeine and Chocolate

Many nursing mothers wonder if it's safe for them to consume coffee, tea, or chocolate. While you may read in herbal books that caffeine-containing substances are "contraindicated" (not recommended) during breastfeeding, this advice is probably way too conservative for most of us.

Caffeine is a naturally occurring plant chemical in green or black tea, coffee, cola drinks, and herbal products containing the South American herb known as guarana. Newborns take longer to break down the caffeine consumed in breast milk because their livers are immature; if your baby is a newborn, be cautious with your use of caffeine. Even if your baby is a few months old, you may find that drinking tea or coffee will leave him wide awake, colicky, or frantic and overstimulated. On the other hand, some babies don't react to caffeine at all. You'll probably be able to gauge just how much caffeine you can drink and at what times of day. Most nursing mothers find that having one or two cups of coffee or tea per day isn't a problem for their babies.

Some babies become colicky or inconsolable when Mom indulges in chocolate (sorry to say). It isn't known what part of chocolate is the culprit, but if your baby is sensitive to chocolate, you will soon know by his colicky behavior. If you're a chocolate lover, it may help to know that as your baby grows he will most likely be less sensitive to what you eat or drink. (Well, most babies that is. You'll just have to find out what's true for your baby.)

You may have to give up chocolate in the early weeks of breastfeeding, but after that, you can probably indulge once in a while. The same holds true for coffee, tea, and other caffeinated products.

something you are eating, try to get to the bottom of it quickly. You can talk to a doctor, lactation specialist, or La Leche League Leader to get more information.

🌿 🌿 🌿

La Leche League has always advocated a diet of whole foods drawn from a wide variety of sources. The wisdom of this advice is more apparent today than ever before. There is, indeed, great value in eating a wide variety of foods in as close to their natural state as possible. This not only gives you a wealth of nutrients but also reduces the amount of artificial ingredients (food colorings, fake flavorings, trans-fats, and a host of unpronounceable chemicals) that you consume. But keep in mind that even if you eat a junk food diet, you can most likely make breast milk that is still far superior in nutrition to any baby formula substitute. Breast milk is still the best you can give.

Because you're feeding your baby the best, you need to make sure that you feed yourself well enough to maintain your own health and energy. Eating a junk food diet will leave you tired and worn out. Take the time to feed yourself adequately. This is your basis of health.

A good diet is the foundation; from there, you'll need exercise, time for yourself, and emotional support from others—plus sleep and more sleep! Allow other people in your life to help take care of you while you take care of your baby, especially during those critical weeks after birth.

$\mathscr{Y}$our Milk Supply

WHEN YOU NEED MORE OR HAVE TOO MUCH

One of the common reasons mothers stop breastfeeding is the often mistaken belief that they aren't making enough milk. In some cases, there may actually be a milk supply problem, but many times it is more a matter of mothers losing confidence because their babies cry a lot, cry after being fed, or want to nurse "frequently." If a mother doubts she is making enough milk and the people around her reinforce the idea by suggesting she should supplement her milk with formula, she may well be on the path to giving up breastfeeding. Perhaps you've experienced a similar problem and you're wondering what to do.

Throughout this chapter, you'll find information on solutions for low milk supply and oversupply. Oversupply? Some nursing mothers have discovered that what they thought was a problem due to a low supply was actually due to too much milk or a too rapid flow. (See "What to Do about Oversupply" later in this chapter.) The good news is there are things you can do about problems with your milk supply, and it's worth taking these steps before discontinuing breastfeeding.

You may find it helpful to review some of the earlier chapters, in particular chapter 1, which discusses the importance of breastfeeding, and chapter 2, which explains some of the basics of nursing and what to expect. Knowing how to tell whether your baby is getting enough milk may reassure you that your supply is just fine. As a very first step, call a breastfeeding helper. This person can help you determine just what sort of a breastfeeding problem you have. Your concerns may very well signal a need to make some adjustments in your breastfeeding routine. La Leche League Leaders and lactation specialists will be responsive to your concerns.

What to Do about Low Milk Supply

You may have heard that low milk supply can be linked to a poor diet, lack of sleep, stress, lack of fluids, a medical condition, or other problems associated with the mother. While this is sometimes the case, low milk supply is more commonly caused by the baby not removing enough milk. Either he isn't latching onto the breast properly, or he isn't breastfeeding often enough.

The early weeks of breastfeeding are critical; this is the time when your milk supply is established based on your baby's nursing patterns. The more milk he removes from the breast, the more milk you make—it's a simple case of supply and demand. If for any reason your baby cannot effectively remove milk, or if he doesn't nurse often enough, your supply of milk will drop. Your supply will stay low if you don't (1) fix the latch so your baby can milk the breast better or (2) increase the number of nursing or pumping sessions per day so that your breasts are stimulated to produce more milk. Until you take these basic steps, all the herbs in the world will not increase your milk supply.

There are herbs that can help you make milk more quickly or help it to flow faster—but they can't address a problem that begins with a poor latch. In fact, many herbalists may be aware of milk supply herbs, but these experts don't necessarily understand the reasons behind a low flow in the first place. I recommend that you consult a breastfeeding expert who can help determine why you're not making enough milk. (La Leche League is a wonderful place to start.) By getting the help of a lactation specialist, you can address any underlying breastfeeding problems while simultaneously working to increase your milk supply. Remember, remedial actions such as herbs can only take you so far. Successful breastfeeding depends primarily on what you and your baby do together.

The following pages include techniques to help increase your milk supply. You can try one or all of them, as needed.

Nurse More Often

Two keys to improving a low supply are removing milk from the breasts frequently through nursing or pumping and making sure that most of the available milk is removed during each session.

You may find that you start producing more milk if you simply let your baby nurse longer at the breast or if you increase the number of breastfeeding sessions per day. Some mothers may need to do both. In the early days and weeks of nursing, babies should breastfeed about every two to three hours, which adds up to eight to twelve times in a twenty-four hour period. If you're pumping your milk, plan on at least eight to twelve sessions per twenty-four hours right from the start, as this most closely mimics how often a baby nurses at the breast. Nursing or pumping at least once a night will help. It is normal for your baby to want to nurse more at night; breastfed babies get about one-third of their milk between midnight and early morning.

Nursing more frequently can improve low supply unless the problem is due to poor latching. If your baby isn't latching onto the breast properly, frequent nursing sessions will only help so much. Your baby may seem to nurse "all the time" but show poor weight gain. If so, find an expert who can help assess the latch. It's possible that your baby looks as if he is latching and suckling correctly but is actually getting little milk for his efforts. A lactation specialist can check how your baby latches to your breast and determine how much milk you are actually producing, as well as help you improve the latch.

Get the Milk Flowing

Regardless of why your milk supply is low, you need to get the milk flowing. You can work on fixing your baby's latch and making sure milk is being removed from your breasts frequently. If your baby isn't on the breast or doesn't nurse effectively, you can keep the milk flowing by expressing it with a pump or by hand. (Note: A baby who is well latched at the breast can get more milk than you can get yourself from a pump or by hand expression, which is why actual nursing sessions are the most productive option.) If the problem is that one breast doesn't make enough milk, focus on increasing the expression of milk on that side. The point is to get the milk out regularly. This will help build or rebuild your supply.

Your baby is the best booster of your milk supply. His suckling stimulates your breasts to make more and more milk. Even if you are expressing your milk by hand or pump, try to find an opportunity to put your baby near the breast. Place him on your chest while you pump; if your baby is willing to nuzzle or lick your breasts, this is a good sign. Any time your baby fusses or shows interest in going to the breast, offer him the chance to nurse. If latching is sometimes a problem, make sure that each latch is as good as possible each time. All of this takes patience and practice. It will help to talk to your breastfeeding supporters (see chapter 2) so they can help you stay focused and encourage you to continue your efforts.

Add More Skin-to-Skin Contact

Increasing skin-to-skin contact with baby has been shown to increase milk production. Skin-to-skin contact means taking off your baby's clothes and placing him next to your bare skin. You can do this in the bath or in bed. Wrap a light blanket over your baby, if needed, to keep both of you warm. You may want to purchase a baby sling for carrying and holding your baby close to you throughout the day. All of this contact not only feels wonderful but also has a purpose: it signals your body to make milk.

Massage the Breasts

Massaging the breasts before breastfeeding or pumping is a time-honored method of increasing the amount of milk flow. Babies who are experienced in nursing at the breast often massage the breasts between their hands during feedings, as they've learned that it makes the milk flow faster.

To increase your milk supply, massage your breasts before nursing or pumping. Lactation consultant Chele Marmet describes useful massage methods in *The Womanly Art of Breastfeeding.* (See appendix A.) Here is a summary of her technique of "massage, stroke, and shake":

1. Massage: Starting at the top of the breast and using a motion similar to breast examination, gently press your fingers into the chest wall and move them in circles on one spot. Don't slide your fingers against the skin; instead, press and massage the tissue underneath. After a few seconds, gently shift your fingers over to a new area of the same breast. Cover the outer sections of the breast first, moving inward and ending up at the areola.

2. Stroke: Next, gently stroke the entire breast from the very top (up by your armpit) down to the nipple. Stroke all around the breast from the outside toward the nipple. This will help you relax and will stimulate the let-down of your milk.

3. Shake: Finally, lean forward and gently shake the breast to help the milk start moving downward.[8]

Do one breast at a time until you get the hang of it. With practice, you may be able to massage both breasts together.

In all circumstances, massage should be gentle. Do not massage your breasts to the point of pain. If you see a practitioner for breast massage, make sure that he or she doesn't hurt your breasts. Ask the practitioner to stop if you feel any pain.

Try Breast Compression

In *The Ultimate Breastfeeding Book of Answers,* pediatrician Jack Newman relates how he observed women in South Africa sometimes squeezing their breasts while nursing their babies. He didn't think about it too much until a woman from South America came to his clinic. He watched as she breastfed her baby, gently squeezing or compressing her breasts as she nursed. Dr. Newman asked why she did this, and she answered that her mother had taught her to do so. In Dr. Newman's own words: "When I asked why her mother had suggested it, she looked at me as if I were from a different planet, and said, 'Because the baby gets more milk.'" [9]

It was then that he realized the connection between breast compression and milk flow. In his book, Dr. Newman explains that compression not only makes the milk flow faster but also helps speed the fatty hind milk out of the breasts, ensuring that the baby gets this richer milk. Drinking this richer milk helps the baby gain weight; at the same time, the breasts are stimulated to make more milk.

If your baby tends to fall asleep at the breast (often a sign of slow milk flow), compression may wake him up and renew his efforts to feed. Following is a synopsis of Dr. Newman's description of breast compression adapted from a patient handout that can be found on the Internet at www.breastfeedingonline.com. (Just click on "Handouts by Jack Newman, MD.") You can learn more about this ancient method by reading Dr. Newman's book or asking a La Leche League Leader.

1. Your baby needs to be latched onto your breast before you start the compressions. To begin, place one hand around your breast, with the thumb on one side of the breast and the fingers on the other side, well back from the areola. Grasp the main body of the breast, not the tip, between your thumb and fingers.

2. Watch your baby nursing. If your baby is well latched and actively nursing in a rhythmic fashion, there is no need to do anything, as the milk is already flowing. Active nursing, according to Dr. Newman,

occurs when your baby is sucking in an "open-pause-close" manner. Your baby opens his jaws, pauses slightly as the milk fills his mouth, and closes his jaws to swallow; he then takes a breath and opens his jaws wide again. You will hear frequent swallowing.

3. Start to compress your breast when your baby starts nibbling or fluttering at the breast—that is, when he no longer swallows frequently. This happens when your milk flow slows down.

4. Squeeze your breast between your fingers and thumb, but not so hard that it hurts. Use gentle, sustained pressure. Your baby should start to suck rhythmically again, with jaws wide open. Keep the pressure on for as long as your baby is actively sucking, then release the pressure and give your hand a rest. Additional milk will probably start to flow when the hand pressure is released. Your baby will often start sucking actively again at this time. Keep watching your baby nurse, and when he starts nibbling again you can resume breast compression.

5. Eventually, the main volume of milk will empty from your breast into your baby's stomach. Once a large volume of milk has been emptied, babies tend to just nibble, even with compression. You can let him nurse a bit longer or offer your other breast now. He may not want it, and that's fine. Or he may take as much again from the second side before becoming satisfied. He may be willing or want to go back to the first side again. You can go back and forth as long as your baby is interested and you are comfortable.*

The key to breast compression is gentle, sustained pressure. Don't squeeze the breasts hard or abruptly, or you may cause yourself some pain. Dr. Newman advises experimenting a bit to see what works for you and your baby. It's not important how you hold your hand on the

*Adapted from Dr. Newman's informative patient handout, "Breast Compression" (handout #15). Copyright © 2003. Used with permission.

breast or apply pressure as long as what you do allows your baby to get more milk. Keep in mind what Dr. Newman says: "You will not always need to do this. As breastfeeding improves, you will be able to let things happen naturally." [10]

Breast Conditions That May Affect Milk Supply

Breast tissue development starts in the teen years when menstruation begins; with each period, more tissue is developed. Pregnancy speeds up the development of breast tissue, and with birth, the breasts are ready to start making milk. But for some women, the milk never comes despite their best efforts and skilled help from others. Inadequate development of the breast tissue may be the cause, although this is rare. It was recently estimated that one in a thousand women have this condition. If you are diagnosed with it, you still may be able to at least partially breastfeed your child.

Milk supply can also be affected by certain hormone-related conditions or by breast reduction or other breast surgeries. Another potential cause of low milk supply is severe and unrelieved engorgement of the breasts, which can damage the milk secretory cells. (Full recovery from such damage may not always be possible.) In these situations, partial breastfeeding may still be possible, especially if an effort is made to increase what milk production there is. Because breastfeeding is healthy for both you and your baby, the effort is worth it.

Dietary/Herbal Help for Low Milk Supply

Some foods have long been considered helpful in increasing milk supply. Grains such as barley, whole grain rice, and oats are especially recommended; in fact, oats have long been given to dairy animals to increase milk supply. These grains are good sources of fiber, choline, calcium, magnesium, and other minerals. They also are rich in beta-glucans, which are now thought to have many health benefits.

Old-fashioned oatmeal, slow-cooked whole grain barley, or other whole-oat preparations are best, though they take longer to prepare. "Instant" oats are more processed and probably won't help your milk supply as much as whole oats. A daily bowl of slow-cooked oatmeal has helped many mothers with their milk supply. (To save time, cook the oats in big batches and heat up a bowl at a time.) Oatmeal cookies and quick breads can also be eaten if porridge doesn't appeal to you.

In Japan, traditional medicine encourages mothers with milk supply problems to eat whole-grain brown rice. Both Chinese and European herbal medicine suggest eating barley. All in all, these grains share several identifiable substances that may work to help regulate your milk supply, without any risk to you or your baby.

Many cultures encourage mothers to eat plenty of dark green vegetables after birth to help with milk production. Adding more green vegetables and fruits to your diet will increase your intake of vitamins, minerals, flavonoids, and fatty acids. Some lactation consultants suggest consuming so-called "green drinks" or "super-green" foods. Many are made with alfalfa and barley greens—plant sources that have been used traditionally to increase milk. Other common ingredients in these products are wheat grass, green algae, and blue-green algae. Blue-green algae is a recent food for humans, so there isn't much traditional information to go on here. If the algae is "wild-crafted" (picked in the wild), be sure that it hasn't been tainted with bird droppings or other contaminants. Note, too, that some brands of "green drinks" contain parsley, an herb that is associated with lowering milk supply. Read the product labels carefully so you can avoid this ingredient.

"Green drinks" can be purchased in powdered form, making them easy to add to other drinks. Cheryl Renfree, a lactation consultant in California, suggests that mothers make a green shake twice a day by adding a scoop of the powdered drink product to soy milk or another beverage; fruits can be added for flavor and additional nutrition. She also recommends adding brewer's yeast for B vitamins, iron, and protein. Many mothers have found brewer's yeast to be helpful not only for building their milk supply but also for combating fatigue, depression, and irritability. "Green drinks" are relatively expensive, but many people swear by them.

Eating select foods may help increase your milk supply, but a nutritious diet does more: it's the foundation for good health. Even if all you do is make an effort to eat fruit with breakfast, add a pile of leafy greens or alfalfa sprouts to your sandwich at lunch, or eat a jumbo serving of vegetables with dinner, you will benefit. These simple steps can go a long way toward preventing fatigue and keeping you energized—which means you'll have more energy for your baby and breastfeeding. A change in diet may be all you need to increase your milk or to find the energy to take on building your supply. See chapter 6 for more on diet.

Taking in enough fluids is important, too. Many mothers sit down to nurse with a water bottle or glass of juice beside them so that they can take frequent sips. In fact, many mothers find that when their milk supply increases, they get thirstier. Drinking to quench your thirst is important, but don't go overboard; drinking more liquids won't produce more milk. In fact, excessive drinking (for example, a gallon a day) may actually suppress milk production. You'll know you're drinking enough fluids if your urine is straw-colored throughout the day. By the way, you do not need to drink milk to make milk. Drink it only if it agrees with you (and your baby).

One of the nice things about herbs is that they can help to increase your milk supply quickly, often making a difference in just a few days' time. Such quick results can be a real morale booster as you work to improve breastfeeding. It's hard work to help a baby improve his latch or to start pumping to supplement the feedings at the breast. Certain herbs can help your body respond to these efforts. Yet, it's important to remember the following about herbal remedies:

- They don't get at the root of a breastfeeding problem, and they won't work unless this underlying problem is addressed.

- They work best when used with all of the basic interventions described earlier in this chapter.

- They can help turn your situation around more quickly, once you've identified the breastfeeding problem and are working to fix it.

- The longer the problem has been going on, the longer it will take to increase your milk supply; but most low-supply problems can be fixed with commitment and perseverance—and the payoff is worth the effort. Plants can be your allies in this endeavor.

Before considering herbs to help you build your milk supply, determine whether you're currently using any herbs that may be limiting or lowering your supply. There have been incidents where moms had a poor supply because they were fond of strong peppermint drops or were using sage lozenges for a sore throat. One mother who had undergone a cesarean birth was taking strong peppermint tea, a helpful remedy after surgery, but the tea prevented her milk from coming in. Her milk quickly increased after she stopped drinking several cups of the tea per day. Check appendix C for more details on herbs that can decrease milk supply.

Herbs that help a low milk supply are known as "galactogogue" herbs. Many lactation specialists consider herbs to be a safe and effective treatment for low milk supply, because herbs usually cause few side effects in the mother or her infant. In very rare situations, babies may develop diarrhea, but the diarrhea usually clears up once the mother reduces her dose or switches to a different herb. Of course, allergy remains a possible risk any time you try a new food or herb. If you have a family history of allergies, stick to herbs that are not known allergens.

Hundreds of plants are used worldwide to increase milk supply, but there are about a dozen in particular that are common in the Western world. This section focuses on those herbs.

Remember: Herbs alone can't solve a breastfeeding problem. Galactogogue herbs may help increase a low milk supply, but the first course of action is to figure out what sort of breastfeeding problem you have. Is it actually a low supply? And if so, what is causing it, and what needs to be done about it?

If you and your breastfeeding helpers determine that you truly do have a low milk supply, it may be helpful to use a medicinal dose of a galactogogue herb. Individual responses will vary; some mothers only need to use an herb for a few days, while a very few mothers may need to continue using herbs for as long as they nurse. Other mothers may not respond to one particular herb but may do very well with another, or with a combination of herbs.

Using Prescription Drugs to Increase Supply

Many practitioners have mothers start with herbs as a first step toward increasing milk supply. Herbs are relatively safe, inexpensive, and easy to get—and all that many mothers will need. Prescription drugs are recommended only when necessary. It helps to know a bit about commonly prescribed drugs so that you can compare your options.

Two prescription drugs are commonly used for increasing supply: metoclopramide and domperidone. Metoclopramide (brand name Reglan) has proven effective in studies and is available in the United States. The drug is familiar to doctors, as they often prescribe it for certain stomach conditions; it increases prolactin levels as a side effect, which makes it useful for low milk supply, especially in the early weeks of breastfeeding. When used for more than two weeks, it may cause depression in some mothers.

The other drug, domperidone, is considered as useful as Reglan and very rarely causes side effects. Domperidone (brand name Motilium) is less familiar to American doctors, as the drug has only orphan status in the United States. This means it's a legal drug, but it isn't manufactured in the United States. Domperidone has been used in Canada and other countries for decades to treat nausea and related stomach conditions, much as metoclopramide is used. Domperidone also raises prolactin, but, unlike metoclopramide, it can't cross into the brain and therefore doesn't cause depression. Because it rarely causes side effects, domperidone can be used for a longer time after birth than metoclopramide. It has also been successfully combined with galactogogue herbs when mothers don't respond to herbal treatments alone.

If you wish to try domperidone, you will need a doctor's prescription. Most lactation consultants and La Leche League Leaders can provide contact information for pharmacies in the United States that can provide domperidone. Take a look at *The Ultimate Breastfeeding Book of Answers* (see appendix A) or other writings by Dr. Jack Newman for more information on this topic.

There are other prescription drugs that also raise prolactin, but these may cause severe side effects.

Appendix C contains specific information about herbs commonly used for low milk supply (see pages 308 through 322); consult this section to become more familiar with each herb and its recommended dose. You'll find profiles of these common galactogogues, including their proper uses, safety, and availability. Although it may seem confusing, I have listed different dosages for some herbs. I did this to give you the range of effective doses that various herbalist lactation consultants have found helpful.

What Is a Medicinal Dose?

A medicinal dose is a large enough quantity of an herb to increase milk. The dose used to stimulate supply is often the same as that taken for other conditions. For a few herbs, though, the dose may be less. Information on effective galactogogue doses is sketchy and sometimes confusing. This is one area where more research is sorely needed.

As you consider which herbs to take, you will also need to think about which form you'd like to take them in: a tincture? a tea? a capsule? a fresh whole herb? It may be helpful to review chapter 4 for information about herbal preparations; the pros and cons of the different forms are discussed in more detail there. If you have a strong preference for a particular herbal preparation—for example, if you enjoy teas—then try that form first and see if it works for you.

From my experience of listening to the wisdom of nursing mothers and lactation specialists, commonly used galactogogue herbs seem to work in any form, so feel free to experiment with several different forms. Many of these herbs do not win prizes for taste, so find the easiest way for you to take them.

Following is a discussion about using galactogogue herbs, arranged by herbal preparation. For more information about any one herb, see the galactogogue herb profiles in appendix C.

Capsules

It's probably fair to say that, of all the galactogogue herbs, fenugreek is the best known in the United States. You'll find recommendations for its use in the writings of Dr. Jack Newman (see appendix A), who states that fenugreek capsules can be used in the early weeks of breastfeeding in a dose of three capsules three times per day to increase milk supply.

Dr. Newman further encourages mothers to take fenugreek with an equal number of blessed thistle capsules. Note that capsule sizes can vary quite a bit; Dr. Newman refers to capsules that weigh about 300–350 mg each. According to Dr. Newman, you can tell that you're taking enough fenugreek when your milk and sweat have the aroma of maple syrup. See the individual herb profiles for fenugreek and blessed thistle in appendix C for more details, including potential side effects. Allergenic and asthmatic patients in particular need to read this material carefully, as both of these herbs can provoke allergy.

Another commonly recommended herb is alfalfa leaf, which is available in tablets and capsules. Alfalfa isn't known to cause allergies; indeed, it is sometimes used to help control allergies. However, alfalfa can cause diarrhea in nursing mothers if started too rapidly, so begin slowly and work your way up to the full dose over a couple of days.

Nettle is another galactogogue herb. Nettle leaf is available in capsules, but this form may not work as well for you as a nettle tincture or tea. Freeze-dried nettle products seem to work best for allergies, but you can try them to see if they increase your milk supply.

Tinctures

Galactogogue herbs can be taken as tinctures. (See chapter 4 for a fuller explanation of tinctures.) Many nursing mothers have found that tinctures are easy to use, though somewhat expensive to buy. Some lactation specialists have noted that mothers seem to respond better to the tinctured herbs than capsules or teas.

Excellent tincture products are available for nursing mothers. A number of companies offer formulas especially for mothers with low milk supply. You can find contact information and dosage recommendations on their company web sites, which are listed in appendix B.

Helpful herbs commonly found in galactogogue tinctures are nettle, fennel, anise, caraway, dill, fenugreek, blessed thistle, vervain, goat's rue, raspberry leaf, hops, and sometimes borage. The herbs are often used in combinations; one popular combination contains blessed thistle, nettle, and fennel. Of all these herbs, goat's rue may be the hardest to find, as it is considered a noxious weed in the United States. (The seed isn't available commercially.) You will probably find it only in specialized breastfeeding tinctures. However, in France, goat's rue has been used since antiquity to build milk and is still commonly used for this purpose.

Not all herbal extracts are the same or work the same for all mothers. If you decide to use a commercial tincture for nursing mothers, keep in mind that tinctures are made with differing concentrations of herbs, water, and alcohol. Also, different products may use different sized droppers and dose descriptions. In general, follow the manufacturer's dose guidelines. Considerable care has gone into adjusting the dose according to the product's effects on milk supply.

Of course, tinctures can be made at home for a fraction of the cost of commercial tinctures. Many herbalists recommend using fresh herbs for tincturing whenever possible. However, seeds can be made into tinctures at any time of the year. Books by herbal experts Rosemary Gladstar and Susun Weed have clear descriptions of how to make herbal tinctures at home. (See appendix A for further information.)

Teas

Teas are one of the oldest and most popular forms of herbal preparation. They are easy to make at home by the cup or by the quart. All you need is a good supply of properly dried herbs. Look for quality herbs available in bulk.

In the following pages, you'll find many recipes for making your own teas, or infusions, which are often a tasty way to get the herbs you need. The recipes use the following herbs and seeds in various combinations: alfalfa, anise, blessed thistle, caraway, coriander, cumin, dill, fennel, fenugreek, goat's rue, hops, marshmallow root, milk thistle, nettle, raspberry leaf, and vervain. More information on these herbs can be found in appendix C.

You might want to add small amounts of other herbs to make these teas taste better. Consider lemon balm, hibiscus, spearmint, lemon verbena, catnip, lemongrass (in small amounts), licorice root (in small amounts), fresh gingerroot, lemon or orange peel, and chamomile. The additional herbs won't interfere with building your milk supply; some are actually considered mild galactogogues. Sweeteners can also make these teas more appealing.

A word to the wise: It has long been suggested that new mothers drink galactogogue teas to "ensure" a good milk supply. Yet, most mothers are capable of making bountiful milk on their own without the help of herbs. (See Chapter 3 for a review of how milk is made.) But if you have a low milk supply, galactogogue teas may be helpful, as long as you take them in adequate amounts. One cup a day usually won't be enough. On the other hand, drinking more than a quart a day may not be wise.

You can mix and match ingredients to see which herbs taste and work the best. If you have allergies, it pays to test individual herbs first by trying a cup of tea made with a single herb and waiting twenty-four hours. We are all unique individuals, and our reactions to these plants will vary.

A Simple Cup of (Medicinal) Tea

In general, use approximately 1 teaspoon of dried herb per teacup (5 oz. or 150 mL) of boiling water. Steep the tea for 10–20 minutes (note that this infusion time is much longer than that needed for a normal cup of tea) and take 2–6 times per day depending on the herb. Keep the tea covered while it steeps. For some herbs, a good tablespoon of the dried herb is needed, so the "teaspoon per teacup" rule is simply a starting point. Exact measures aren't that important for most of these herbs, but check an herb's profile in appendix C to be sure. If the taste is too strong, you can add more hot water after steeping. The single-cup method is best for aromatic seeds such as fennel and anise, for cold infusions of marshmallow, and for hops, which is best taken in small single doses.

A Quart of Tea at a Time: The Standard Quart Infusion

Lactation specialists have found that starting with a relatively high dose of herbs seems to kick-start milk production. If you make a quart at a time, you can whip up a day's supply all at once. The quart will give you a strong dose of herbs that can be conveniently sipped throughout the day. Canning quart jars are good for brewing the tea as they hold a day's supply, will not break when boiling water is added, and have tight lids.

To make a standard quart infusion, use 1 oz. of dried herbal material per quart or liter of water. A dry ounce weighs about 30 g. Use a kitchen scale to measure the herbs. If you do not have a scale, you can use these rough substitute measures: an ounce of leafy herbs is about 2 handfuls; an ounce of seeds is 2–4 tablespoons (depending on the density of the seeds). Use the seed weight conversion table on page 125 to determine how many tablespoons of a given seed are in an ounce. Place the herbs in a quart jar and cover with boiling water. Or place the herbs in cold water and bring to a boil, then immediately pour into a quart jar. Cover, steep, and strain. Avoid copper, aluminum, or plastic containers. Do not microwave herbs.

Steeping time varies from herb to herb. Blessed thistle, vervain, and especially goat's rue are very bitter. When using these herbs by themselves, steep no more than 20–30 minutes, then strain. Use small amounts when steeping overnight with more pleasant tasting herbs. (For additional strategies, see pages 123 through 126.) Nettle and alfalfa, on the other hand, do not go bitter and will have more mineral content if steeped overnight. The delicate, volatile oils of aromatic seeds are easily lost; keep tightly covered and steep no more than 20–30 minutes before straining. Prepared tea should be kept refrigerated. A cup may be sipped cold or, better, gently heated first. The volume of tea after straining is your maximum daily dose. Do not drink it all at once. Instead, drink it in 3 or more doses throughout the day. As your milk production increases, typically within 2–4 days, you'll probably find that you can reduce the dose or even discontinue using the tea altogether.

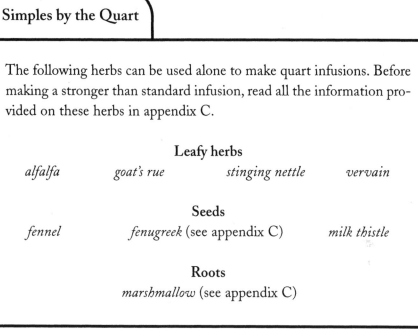

Simples by the Quart

The following herbs can be used alone to make quart infusions. Before making a stronger than standard infusion, read all the information provided on these herbs in appendix C.

Leafy herbs

alfalfa   *goat's rue*   *stinging nettle*   *vervain*

Seeds

fennel   *fenugreek* (see appendix C)   *milk thistle*

Roots

marshmallow (see appendix C)

Making Your Own Blend

An herb can be used by itself to make a tea, or infusion, or it can be combined with other herbs. It's easy to make your own custom blends once you know how to go about mixing the herbs. Experiment to find combinations that work best for you and taste good. Some herbs are best used in combinations (e.g., hops, raspberry leaves), and many herbs make a better tasting tea if combined with sweet aromatic seeds.

To prepare a blend or recipe for tea that combines aromatic seeds and other herbs, simply add a quart of boiling water to 1 oz. of the mixed herbs and steep for 20–30 minutes. Or, make a standard quart infusion using 1 oz. of your choice of leafy herbs. Gently heat 1 cup

Making Your Own Blend

(5–8 oz.) of this prepared tea, add 1–3 teaspoons of freshly crushed aromatic seeds (mixed to taste), and tightly cover for 10-15 minutes. This is probably the better method for combining leafy herbs and delicate aromatic seeds.

Measurements

"Handfuls" are often used by herbalists for measuring dried leaves and flowers. One handful is approximately 2/3 of a cup by volume.

Measuring plant parts (for 1 oz. of herb):

chopped leaves	2 handfuls of chopped-up dried leaves
whole leaves	3 handfuls of dried whole leaves
flowers	2 big handfuls of dried, crumbled flowers
seeds	2–4 tablespoon seeds, depending on the seed

Leaves:

When used in combination, some herbs make up a larger proportion of the mix (e.g., stinging nettle) than others (e.g., hops). Use the rough proportions below to make your own blends.

alfalfa (larger amounts)

blessed thistle (moderate amounts)

goat's rue (small to moderate amounts; disagreeably bitter)

hops (small amounts only)

raspberry (moderate amounts, but don't use long-term)

stinging nettle (larger amounts)

vervain (moderate amounts)

Roots:

Use root pieces or small amounts of powdered root in blends. If you are going to use marshmallow root, read its profile in appendix C first to

Making Your Own Blend

prevent a gooey mess. Instructions for making cold infusions and decoctions and suggestions for using them in tea blends are given there.

Seeds, freshly crushed:
See the table below for converting seed weights to tablespoons. Crush the seeds after measuring and just before preparing the tea.

anise	caraway	coriander	cumin
dill	fennel	fenugreek	milk thistle

Seed weights in tablespoons:

1 tablespoon of seed	grams	tablespoon per ounce
anise	10.5	3
caraway	10.5	3
coriander	6.9	4
cumin	8	3–4
dill	7	4
fennel	7.5	3–4
fenugreek (whole)	14	2
fenugreek (ground)	10	3
milk thistle	10.5	3

An example of making your own blend

Let's say you like the taste of stinging nettle but would also like to include blessed thistle in your blend. You can make a mix using a smaller amount of blessed thistle than stinging nettle (maybe 1 part blessed thistle and 4 parts stinging nettle). Mix 1 handful of blessed thistle for every 4 handfuls of stinging nettle. To make tea, use 1 oz. (2 handfuls) of the mixture per quart of boiling water and steep, overnight if you wish. If you find the tea too bitter, steep for a shorter time or use less blessed thistle. Or you may decide to offset the bitterness by adding fennel seed to the leaf mix. To do

Making Your Own Blend

so, use less of the leaf mix and add the fennel seed. The seed weight conversion table shows that it takes 3–4 tablespoons of fennel seed to make an ounce. To make your quart of tea, then, you would use 1/2 oz. (1 handful) of leaves and 1/2 oz. (about 2 tablespoons) of fennel seed, freshly crushed. Or you could brew the blessed thistle and stinging nettle leaf mixture separately (steeping the nettle overnight to extract more minerals, while steeping the blessed thistle for 20 minutes to control bitterness). Combine, then add about a heaping spoonful of fennel seed to each individual cup of tea you make.

If you would prefer to follow recipes, you may want to try one or more of the following. For some recipes, no exact amount of the herb is given—only a list of herbs that have been traditionally combined. You can make these blends using about equal weights of leafy herbs to seeds. In all cases, no more than about an ounce of herbs in total are used per quart infusion. The daily dose of tea is unchanged: no more than a quart of the infusion per day.

Mumma's Milk Tea

This traditional recipe of midwives can be dry mixed ahead of time and made a cup at a time. It is always best to crush aromatic seeds just before use. Experiment with different proportions of the leaf and seed herbs.

alfalfa	*blessed thistle*	*fennel seed*
marshmallow	*stinging nettle*	*vervain*

Milch-Building Tea

This recipe comes from Germany.

anise seed   *caraway seed*   *goat's rue*
stinging nettle   *vervain*

Tasty Tea

This is a particularly tasty recipe! Pour 1 cup of boiling water over the seeds and steep for 15–20 minutes.

1 teaspoon cumin seed   1 teaspoon dill seed   1 teaspoon fennel seed

Susun Weed is a traditional herbalist and the author of three terrific books on women's herbs. The following two recipes are reprinted with permission from her popular book *Wise Woman Herbal for the Childbearing Year*, published by Ash Tree Publishing. I like the fennel/barley water recipe especially. Try barley water as a base for other seed teas, such as dill seed. Dill seed tea, when taken by the mother, can help with a baby's colic.

Susun Weed's Fennel/Barley Water Tea

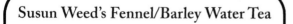

1/2 cup barley (regular, pearled)   1 teaspoon fennel seed

Soak barley in 3 cups cold water overnight, or boil for 25 minutes. Strain barley and save for soup; refrigerate barley water. Heat 1–2 cups barley water to boiling as needed. Pour over fennel seed, and steep no longer than 30 minutes.

Susun Weed's Nursing Formula

1 oz. blessed thistle or borage leaves (dried)
1 oz. raspberry or stinging nettle leaf (dried)
1 teaspoon aromatic seeds

Place leaves in a half-gallon jar and fill to the top with boiling water. Cap tightly and let steep overnight. Strain and refrigerate liquid. As you get ready to nurse, heat 1 cup of brew to near boiling. Pour over 1 teaspoon of any of these aromatic seeds:

anise	*caraway*	*coriander*
cumin	*dill*	*fennel*

Let the tea brew and cool for 5 or more minutes before drinking.

Note: Some have sounded cautions about using borage leaf while nursing, due to the presence of the potentially toxic pyrrolizidine alkaloids in the leaf. (These alkaloids are not present in the seed oil.) However, borage leaf has very tiny amounts of this toxin. Still, you may want to use less controversial herbs or limit how much borage you consume. Fresh borage leaves taste like cucumber, and I enjoy them as a salad garnish (but not too often and not too much).

Mega-galactogogue Tea

Many mothers have found that using herbs right from the start can be helpful in establishing a good milk supply. One mother experienced a low milk supply with her first baby, a problem that she couldn't overcome

Mega-galactogogue Tea

at the time, even with excellent breastfeeding help. She decided that she never wanted to go through that experience again, so during her next pregnancy she started using the galactogogue herbs while pregnant and continued using them after giving birth. The second time around she found success. Here's what she did in her own words:

Prenatal: I used a healthy handful of this mix: equal portions of red raspberry leaf and nettle, with slightly smaller portions of alfalfa and red clover blossom. I'd use a heaping handful in about a quart of almost boiling water, mix, and steep overnight. (Yes, I made it strong and usually drank it iced.)

Postpartum: Used the same basic formula postpartum, but leaned a little heavier on the nettle. Added hops flower, blessed thistle, marshmallow root (all in about equal portions, about a handful), fenugreek powder (a heaping teaspoon per quart) and goat's rue powder (a heaping teaspoon per quart). Same deal—used a large handful of the herb mix and added the powders to about a quart of water and steeped till cool. Drink a quart a day—tastes pretty bitter but is okay iced, once you get used to it. I started drinking it within an hour after birth! (I had it mixed up ahead of time in preparation.)

A note of caution: Although raspberry leaf may initially increase milk supply, its astringency may subsequently decrease it. Use of red clover blossoms during pregnancy is somewhat controversial, as they may increase bleeding during labor and delivery. Most mothers do not need to use herbs right from birth to make enough milk. This woman had specific reasons for doing so. Before using the mega-galactogogue preparations above, talk to an herbal expert you trust.

Teas and Taste

If you really hate the taste of the herbs used in these recipes, consider adding small amounts of spearmint, orange peel, lemon peel, lemongrass, chamomile, or other tasty herbs to your mixtures. Just don't use peppermint, as it can decrease your milk supply. Adding sweetener can also make many herbs more palatable—especially the bitter ones.

Tips for Sustaining Your Supply

A few nursing mothers discover that they cannot sustain their milk supply without the continued use of herbal remedies. If you find yourself in this situation, you may want to "rotate" your use of herbs. Sometimes, herbs lose their effectiveness after a couple of weeks. Another good reason for rotating is that the long-term use of large doses of herbs increases the risk of adverse effects. (The same is true with drugs.) You can switch to another herb for a time, then go back to the previous one later, if you wish. For example, some nursing mothers have noted that stopping their use of fenugreek after several weeks and then restarting after a week's hiatus seems to renew its benefits. Each woman is unique and responds to herbs differently.

Mothers who have severe milk supply problems sometimes get a more sustained response when alternating between various single and combination tinctures. You could, for example, use a simple form of a tincture until your response to it slackens, and then switch to a combination tincture for a while. For some women, switching preparations in this way seems to reinvigorate milk production. Be sure to keep in touch with your breastfeeding helpers as you try different options.

What Traditional Chinese Medicine (TCM) Can Offer

Traditional Chinese Medicine, or TCM, has developed remedies to relieve many postpartum conditions, including low milk supply. TCM practitioners gather clues from both mother and baby, viewing the two as a dyad. (See chapter 3 for an explanation of the dyad.) Diagnosis and treatment are individualized for the dyad. TCM practitioners use various approaches to treat low milk supply, including moxibustion, acupuncture, dietary changes, and herbs. Chinese medicinal literature suggests a number of types and combinations of medicinal plants for treating low milk supply. Which ones work best depend on the practitioner's diagnosis for that mother and child.

To take full advantage of this system of medicine, it is best to see a TCM practitioner before attempting to use a TCM remedy on your own. TCM practitioners have an amazingly sophisticated knowledge of how herbs work together, and they are generally confident about being able to help mothers with low milk supply. If you are interested in Chinese remedies, see a reputable TCM practitioner for an individualized diagnosis and treatment plan. (See chapter 5 for more on TCM.)

What to Do about Oversupply

Mothers are usually blessed with an abundant milk supply as soon as the milk comes in after birth. With a good latch (which helps the baby to control the flow of milk and keeps the mother's nipples from getting sore), feedings go smoothly and the baby thrives. But, as many mothers know, it can sometimes take a bit of work to get to this point. The baby may struggle at the breast, choke with the let-down of milk, or pull off from the breast soon after let-down. The baby may spit up a lot of milk, or have a green, frothy stool, or suffer bouts of unexplained crying (sometimes mistaken for colic). Naturally, his mother may wonder if something is wrong with her milk, or worry that there isn't enough milk to satisfy her baby.

As it turns out, many of these difficulties seen in the early weeks may be related to an oversupply instead of a low supply. For many women, the let-down or milk-ejection reflex is stronger when there is a lot of milk in the breast. The rapid flow of milk that follows isn't easily handled by the baby, who may pull off from the breast when the flow is strong. An abundant let-down or a too-rapid milk flow can also cause the baby to choke, spit up, and cry during feedings. He may refuse to settle into a feed, or he may nurse for only very short periods of time.

If your baby is a vigorous nurser, seems very alert, is gaining weight well, and yet still seems to be struggling at the breast in some way, talk to your breastfeeding helpers about the situation. (See chapter 2 for more on breastfeeding support.) There are many potential solutions to your problem, but it's best to have early help from a breastfeeding expert who can assess your situation and help you figure out what to do.

If allowed to continue, oversupply and a strong let-down can result in the baby turning away from the breast as a source of comfort. He may nurse less frequently or for shorter periods of time, or he may refuse to nurse at all, particularly if given a bottle (whose flow he can control). Less nursing at the breast can result in a low milk supply. Mothers in this situation may find that taking steps to move the milk from their breasts (see "What to Do about Low Milk Supply" earlier in this chapter), coupled with helping herbs, will quickly reverse the supply problem. If you're in this situation, seek the skilled aid of a lactation expert.

Here are some general steps that can be taken if you are in the early weeks of breastfeeding and your supply is "too much, too fast" for your baby. Your breastfeeding helper may check:

- The baby's latch: A better latch may help him to better control the flow of milk. A poor latch may leave the baby choking after being flooded with milk.

- The baby's position: He may do better when positioned with his head higher than your breast, so he doesn't choke so much. Make use of gravity to help the milk flow into his stomach.

- How you nurse: Switching your baby frequently from breast to breast during a feeding session can create problems. If your baby is moved off the breast before he can get to the rich hind milk, he will get a double dose of the watery foremilk. (With its high lactose content, the foremilk can ferment in his bowel, causing cramps.) The solution is simple. First, allow your baby to finish at the first side at his own pace. Once he has either fallen asleep or taken himself off the breast, burp him and offer him the other breast. If this doesn't improve things, offer the same breast several sessions in a row before allowing baby to nurse from the other side. (Some mothers find that they need to nurse their baby exclusively on one breast in the morning, and on the other in the afternoon.) If the breast that your baby isn't nursing from becomes engorged, express a small amount of milk to relieve the discomfort. As the supply slows down, the engorgement will pass.

- Frequency of nursing sessions: If you go a long time between sessions and your baby wakes up ravenous, he will vigorously latch on; this can stimulate a very strong let-down and a more rapid flow of milk. Avoiding long periods between nursing sessions can help. Watch for your baby's signs of hunger—eye movements, small sounds, body movements—and act on them quickly. Frequent feedings also increase the fat content of the milk, which helps babies who have frothy stools or who aren't gaining weight.

- Draining of the breasts: Emptying one breast at a feeding will slow the overall stimulation of your milk supply, as discussed above. Nursing on one side and leaving the other breast full for longer slows the rate of milk synthesis. Don't short-circuit this by pumping extra milk; this will stimulate the breasts to fill more quickly again.

An overly abundant milk supply can cause sore nipples, plugged ducts, mastitis, thrush, nipple blanching, and breast pain. Contacting a lactation specialist or another breastfeeding helper is essential. Often, slowing down the milk production can help these problems clear up, but you may need the guidance of an expert. Chapter 8 includes information about breast problems and what you can do about them.

Sometimes, an abundant supply or forceful let-down doesn't respond to the usual interventions, or a problem with oversupply returns. In cases like these, expert help is needed. Talk to your breast-feeding helpers to see if you can get to the root of the problem. Be sure to mention any medications, vitamins, herbs, or other dietary supplements you may be using. It's possible that these products are causing an increase in your milk supply. Sometimes, mothers unknowingly use galactogogue herbs that stimulate their milk supply or strengthen their let-down. Discontinuing these herbs allows the mothers to resolve their oversupply problem more rapidly. If you tend toward oversupply, watch out for galactogogues; you may be responsive to even small doses of the more powerful ones. (Appendix C lists common herbs and notes which are galactogogues.)

Herbal Remedies for Oversupply

Just as there are herbs for low milk supply, there are herbs for oversupply. A number of herbs have been used around the world for this purpose—peppermint, sage, and parsley being among the best. Because they work against milk production, they are called "antigalactogogues."

Traditionally used for weaning (see chapter 11), peppermint, sage, and parsley have also proven themselves effective for taming an over-abundant milk supply. Even if you use these herbs, however, you will need to take the basic steps recommended for slowing milk production. Do not rely on herbs alone. The effective dose of an herb varies from mother to mother. For some, a very small dose is sufficient. For others, a larger dose is required. In any case, use an herb only as long as you need it. Progress is often seen within a week, and over this period of time less and less of the herb should be needed.

Herbs and Oversupply: Two Stories

It isn't uncommon for herbs to have the unintended effect of increasing a mother's milk supply enough to cause a problem. Following are two stories about how this can happen.

I was asked to assist a mother who had recurring plugged milk ducts that had repeatedly led to mastitis. The mother had had the same problem when her baby was a newborn, and, at that time, she realized it was related to an overabundant milk supply, which she fixed. But now her baby was several months old, and breastfeeding had been going smoothly until this point. We discussed all the medications and herbal remedies she was using; she said she had recently started taking alfalfa tablets (15 per day) to help with her allergies. Alfalfa is a galactogogue, and she was using a medicinal dose. Together, we realized that her plugged ducts were related to her overabundant milk supply. Once she stopped taking the alfalfa, she was free of plugged ducts and had no return bouts of mastitis.

On another occasion, a La Leche League Leader called me about a mother of a very colicky baby. She had been trying to help the colic by drinking fennel seed tea. While it's true that nursing mothers can drink fennel tea (or teas made with anise, caraway, or dill seed) for colic relief, in this case, it wasn't helping. The baby was choking and struggling at the breast. The mother hadn't realized that fennel can cause a stronger let-down of milk. Ironically, the baby became more colicky from the very measures his mother took to help the colic. The mother's otherwise admirable approach to treating colic didn't get to the root of the problem, which, in this case, was probably related to oversupply or frequent switching at the breast.

Before taking any of these antigalactogogues, it is essential to talk to a breastfeeding expert. You·need to know for sure if your breastfeeding problem is truly a matter of an overabundant supply. It's possible to overdo herbs and end up having to rebuild your milk supply. If you are interested in using an herbal remedy, share the information in this book with your lactation specialist. The information here is based on the experiences of many herbalist lactation specialists who have worked with mothers in oversupply.

Some information about the antigalactogogues peppermint, sage, and parsley follows.

Peppermint: Some forms of peppermint are more effective at reducing milk supply than others. Peppermint tea, for example, isn't known to be able to lower an overabundant milk supply, probably because it doesn't contain enough menthol. Mothers with oversupply and a very strong let-down tend to need the more concentrated peppermint essential oil, which has a higher menthol content. Strong peppermint candies eaten frequently throughout the day have helped some mothers, according to Lisa Marasco, IBCLC. You may wish to make a cup of peppermint tea and add several drops to a quarter teaspoon of essential oil or spirits of peppermint immediately before drinking it. Some nursing mothers may need to drink several cups of this remedy per day.

Do not use peppermint essential oil if you are prone to heartburn or have gastric reflux disease. Instead, try enteric-coated peppermint capsules, which pass through the stomach before release (although these capsules can be pricey). Women with gallbladder or liver disease should consult a doctor or knowledgeable healthcare provider before using peppermint. The herb has been used to treat biliary tract disease, but it can worsen the condition if misused. Side effects from large doses of peppermint oil are rare; still, it is prudent to watch for a skin rash, slowed heart rate, or muscle tremor. However, the amounts used for oversupply would not be expected to cause these symptoms.

Sage: This herb is almost legendary for lowering milk supply, and, among herbalists, it is the most widely recognized herb to use for weaning. A note of caution: Never use sage essential oil; taken internally it has caused seizures. Use only powdered or coarsely cut leaves (such as the ones you can buy in a grocery store), and use the least amount for the shortest period of time. Keep in mind that powdered leaves are only potent for one month, while the coarsely cut leaves are good for eighteen months.

Although sage isn't considered toxic, the leaves do contain thujone, a toxic substance. Some other plants that contain thujone, such as wormwood, are considered toxic, but, for some reason (perhaps a mix of different plant chemicals), sage leaves do not have a toxic effect when used by humans. To decrease milk, small doses of sage may be taken for a few days. Such usage has not been associated with toxic reactions in mothers or their children. Native American healers use other types of plants that are commonly called sage (for example, sweet sage) to help slow milk, but these herbs are used with some risk, as they also contain thujone and little is known about their toxicity.

If you don't like the taste of sage, try this innovative suggestion from Sharon Knorr, IBCLC: Make a peanut butter and honey sandwich, then open up one corner and put the powdered sage just inside. Close up the sandwich and start eating on that corner to get it over with. Peanut butter and honey do a fair job of disguising the taste of sage. Something fruity to drink with the sandwich helps, too.

The dose of sage needed to tame oversupply will vary, although usually about 1 tablespoon of sage is needed to make a cup of tea or broth (which is tastier). Steep the infusion for 10–15 minutes, and drink 3–6 times per day.

Sage is also tinctured. Follow the label directions scrupulously, as the strength of tinctures varies from manufacturer to manufacturer. Do not use tinctures or large doses for more than a week or so at a time, as adverse reactions may occur. Also, be aware that slowing milk production can make you more fertile.

Sage is used for many conditions, often in smaller doses than that used for reducing supply. Generally, overdose symptoms are seen only if more than 3–4 tablespoons of the powdered leaf are taken at a time; otherwise, dose-related adverse reactions are unlikely, even in the amounts commonly used for oversupply. Dizziness, rapid heart rate, and hot flashes may develop when sage leaf is used for too long or in overdose. Watch for these reactions and discontinue use if they occur.

Parsley: Parsley leaf is used to lower milk supply; however, the essential oil is toxic and should not be used.

More than one mother has reported that her milk supply took a big dip after feasting on tabbouleh for several days. (Tabbouleh salad is about half parsley.) Similarly, mothers have noticed that drinking parsley juice or taking parsley juice tablets reduced their supply of milk.

To deliberately lower milk supply using parsley, you'll probably need quite a large quantity of the herb. Dried parsley capsules can be used, but you may need to take a lot of them: about 12 capsules each day (4 capsules, 3 times per day). Do not use parsley in large amounts if you have inflammatory kidney disease, however. Parsley may not be the first herb to try for severe oversupply situations. But if you're already using other herbs for oversupply, adding liberal amounts of parsley to the mix can only help.

Another remedy that shouldn't be overlooked is cabbage leaves (or ice—your choice), which can be applied to your breasts to prevent or reduce engorgement during the time when you're trying to reduce your milk supply. Discontinue the use of the cabbage leaves as your situation improves. Some nursing mothers have reported that drinking carrot juice in the morning helps damp down an abundant milk supply. Another option is sorrel, which can be eaten in small amounts; however, sorrel contains oxalates, which can irritate the stomach and kidneys.

Over-the-counter preparations containing pseudoephedrine (the active ingredient in Sudafed) have been successfully used by lactation consultants to help suppress milk supply. But the herbs mentioned here may be more pleasant to use, as pseudoephedrine can overstimulate you, or even your baby.

One note of caution: Some suggest rubbing camphor or menthol creams on the breast. Avoid these remedies, as your baby could suffer breathing difficulties while nursing.

🌿 🌿 🌿

When it comes to milk supply, looks can be deceiving. What may appear to be a problem of too little milk can actually be the opposite. Always follow one crucial rule when you think you may have a problem with your milk supply: Talk to a lactation specialist before trying to treat the problem yourself. Keep in close touch with this specialist while you're working to adjust your supply. And watch your baby for clues. He will let you know when things improve.

Breastfeeding experts can do so much more than simply recommend an herb. They can help correct an underlying breastfeeding problem that you may not be aware of. It is essential to get help. The information in this book cannot replace individualized evaluation by an expert. Working with someone who is dedicated to helping you nurse will provide critical emotional support for your struggle while helping you and your baby to breastfeed successfully.

$\mathscr{B}$reast Problems

I remember feeling rather smug and blissful for the first couple of days after my daughter was born. We had made great strides with breast-feeding. I nursed my daughter at least every two hours around the clock, managing to keep my breasts relatively empty. Yes, my nipples were a bit sore—I was applying gobs of lanolin to them after every nursing session—but at least I had escaped engorgement. Surely, nothing could make my breasts swell. By day three, however, my breasts began to get firm within an hour of breastfeeding. It was clear that, despite my furious nursing, my milk wasn't going out as fast as it was coming in.

By day four, my breasts felt like they were bursting, and my nipples developed cracks and scabs. Although my dear "barracuda" daughter was doing a whole lot of sucking and nursing, she wasn't latching correctly. Nursing her frequently hydrated her well enough, but she wasn't taking out all of the milk that she could have. This was the main cause for the engorgement and my discomfort.

I knew it was time to get out *The Womanly Art of Breastfeeding,* a book I was sure could help me. I reviewed the sections on positioning a baby for breastfeeding and latching properly. I decided to use pillows to help get my daughter up to my breast level; she had been sliding down my areola, hanging on tightly to the nipple. I cut way back on my use of lanolin, as it was causing my daughter to slip down onto the tip of the nipple while she nursed. I took a pain medication that my doctor assured me was safe to use while nursing. I then had a lovely hot shower, soaking off all the scabs, and immediately afterwards nursed my daughter. That nursing session was the one that finally relieved some of the engorgement. I focused on improving her latch, and, within hours, the engorgement was manageable. Two days later, my nipples were no longer sore and the healing was complete.

What amazes me to this day is how these challenges—engorgement, sore nipples, difficulty latching—were all related. It was like a puzzle; figuring out how the pieces fit together led to the solution. In my case, focusing on the important issue of latching helped resolve the other problems I was experiencing.

Like many nursing mothers, I felt completely overwhelmed when I experienced breast problems so early on. It's easy to see how any mother can become discouraged, especially in the early days of breastfeeding. There is good news, though: Fixing a latching problem can often solve many other breastfeeding problems, too. With patience, persistence, and perhaps the help of an expert, you can soon get back on track.

Engorgement

While your breasts may seem enormous during pregnancy, they will probably get even bigger after birth when your milk comes in. At some point between the second and sixth day after your baby is born, your milk will automatically become much more plentiful. Up until that time, your baby will get colostrum while nursing, and this miraculous substance supplies him with all the nutrition he needs during those early days. Your breasts will probably feel quite full when your milk comes in—perhaps almost to "bursting." This is due to the extra blood that is drawn to your breasts, followed by the normal swelling of breast tissue as it gears up for high milk production. Usually, the swelling subsides in a few days if you nurse frequently.

However, for some mothers the swelling leads to engorgement, as it did for me. Engorgement may occur even if you have done everything "right," although, in most cases, when the baby is properly latched, frequent nursing sessions in the first few days will prevent severe engorgement.

If you become engorged, you may awaken to discover achy breasts that feel almost "rock hard." You may even run a low-grade fever. Not only is engorgement painful, but it can also flatten the nipples and areola, making it more difficult for your baby to latch properly. This can lead to an even greater backup of milk, which, in turn, can lead to plugged milk ducts and mastitis.

To fix a nursing problem you must figure out how it began in the first place. In my case, it was the result of a poor latch. Once the latch was fixed, nursing sessions were more productive and the engorgement subsided. If you become engorged, be ready to take action quickly so the engorgement doesn't get worse. Seek the help of a La Leche League Leader or other lactation specialist right away. It is critical to address the problem quickly. With help, you can avoid the need to supplement with formula and won't be tempted to give up breastfeeding.

As you work to find solutions, continue nursing so that your baby gets enough breast milk and your breasts stay softer and more comfortable. If your baby is having trouble latching, you can express some milk by hand or with a pump to soften your breasts. Try not to wait too long between nursing sessions, however; in the first week or so of breastfeeding, your baby may want to nurse at least every two or three hours. Your baby may want to nurse even more frequently if he is not getting a good, deep latch. Once the latch is effective, he can take larger volumes of milk at a time and will probably go a bit longer before nursing again. Have patience until then and throw away the clock.

An Engorgement Solution: One Woman's Story

Eleanor experienced severe engorgement back in the days when babies were kept in the hospital nursery and brought out only every four hours for feedings. At that time, many nurses at Eleanor's hospital disapproved of mothers who chose to breastfeed, and they wouldn't cooperate with her desire to have the baby brought to her more frequently. Needless to say, her breasts were bursting with milk and she was in great pain. An English nurse who came on duty took one look at Eleanor and went into action. First, the nurse filled a large basin with very cold water. Alongside of it, she filled another large basin with hot water (not burning, but comfortably hot). Then she took Eleanor to the hot basin and plunged her breasts deep into the water; just as Eleanor relaxed into the feeling, the nurse moved her to the cold water and had her dip her breasts in it. Just when Eleanor couldn't stand the cold any longer, she went back to the hot water. This back-and-forth action continued a couple more times, then, all of a sudden, Eleanor's milk was spraying everywhere. Her let-down reflex had kicked in, and the engorgement was on its way to being relieved. The baby was brought in to breastfeed, and the helpful nurse saw to it that the baby latched on correctly. Although breastfeeding had gotten off to a rocky start, things were certainly looking up.

Medically speaking, Eleanor received a contrast sitz bath. This is an old but helpful method of stimulating circulation in body tissues. It is very useful for swollen, sore bottoms, too. See chapter 6 on postpartum care for more on sitz baths.

Helping the Milk Move Out

The best way to relieve engorgement is to get the milk flowing, and the quickest way to get the milk flowing is to nurse a baby who is willing and able to breastfeed. In some cases, however, a baby may not be able to nurse, or may be not be available to nurse (if, for example, he is receiving medical care in the hospital). If this is the case, you may need to remove milk from your breasts using either hand expression or a breast pump. (Call on a lactation specialist for help, or read La Leche League's *The Womanly Art of Breastfeeding* for further information.) Hand-expression and pumping are both learned skills, and it can take a few practice sessions before you get much milk for your efforts. It can sometimes be hard to let down for a pump. Yet, you need a let-down (also called a milk-ejection reflex) to get the milk to flow.

Below is a list of techniques for stimulating let-down. They can be helpful whether you are hand-expressing, pumping, or nursing your baby directly. (See "An Engorgement Solution: One Woman's Story" on page 144 for a nearly forgotten method for stimulating let-down.)

- Ask someone to gently rub your back.

- Take a warm shower before nursing or expressing your milk.

- Gently massage your breasts before nursing, hand-expressing, or pumping. This can make the let-down happen faster.

- Bathe your breasts in warm water so you can massage them even more gently. Make the bathwater slippery by adding a handful of marshmallow root powder (sold in bulk at natural food stores). The marshmallow root may have a medicinal action on the let-down, too. Other soothing, slippery baths can be made with rolled oats, oat flour, or slippery elm. Slosh the slippery mixture on your breasts and gently rub them. This may trigger a let-down on the spot. If this occurs, let the milk flow into the basin or catch it in a clean container. Nurse your baby or express your milk immediately afterwards.

- If you're having persistent problems with a slow let-down, ask a knowledgeable herbalist about using black cohosh, which can help trigger the let-down response. Only a few doses are needed in most cases. There are no reports of adverse effects in infants with the maternal use of black cohosh after birth. Some women may be sensitive or allergic to black cohosh, however. Black cohosh is used with difficult births, where the powers of labor have slowed. It has been used to assist delivery of the placenta and to keep the uterus well contracted. Black cohosh was also traditionally used by the Iroquois to treat breastfeeding problems. These uses indicate that black cohosh may have an oxytocin-like effect or assist the body's use of oxytocin. (Oxytocin is the hormone that signals the breast to release, or let down, milk.) Such actions would explain why this herb helps improve let-down problems. Research about herbs and oxytocin is sorely lacking, so it is best to get expert help when considering its use.

External Remedies

External remedies include poultices, compresses, and plasters. A poultice consists of fresh plant material (or dried plant material that has been moistened) placed directly over the affected area, such as a wound or swelling. Poultices are often held in place with a wet dressing covered with a dry bandage. A compress is a clean cloth dipped in plain water, herbal tea, a decoction, vinegar, or a tincture and placed on the skin. You can also make a compress by enclosing the wet herbal material in a cloth. Plasters are sticky preparations thinly spread on a dry covering cloth and applied to the body (for example, a mustard plaster).

You may not need to take out much milk to soften the areola enough for your baby to latch on well. But if your baby cannot latch (for whatever reason), any milk you express should be fed to your baby with a cup or spoon. Expressing milk can relieve some of your pain *and* is needed to encourage your breasts to keep making milk. (Yes, your breasts are trying to make a lot of milk, which accounts for all the extra fluid and swelling.)

If no milk is removed during engorgement, the body quickly gets the message that there is no baby and stops producing milk. It cannot be overstated that getting the milk moving within that first week is the key to preventing milk supply problems down the road. In addition, the frequent removal of milk helps prevent plugged ducts, inflammation, and other consequences of pressure in the breasts. And, of course, feeding your baby with your milk avoids the need to feed him formula.

With painful engorgement, you may be tempted to apply heat packs to your breasts to ease the pain. But heat isn't recommended because it may worsen the engorgement by bringing even more fluid to the breasts or increasing tissue swelling. You can take a warm shower or bathe your breasts in warm water right before nursing, however. In fact, warm compresses—dry or wet—applied just before nursing are very relaxing and can help get the milk flowing. For pain and swelling, it is recommended that you use cabbage leaves (see "Cabbage, Herbs, and Anti-inflammatory Agents" later in this chapter) or ice packs on the breasts in between nursing sessions. Just before you breastfeed, remove the packs and apply warmth, if desired, to help with let-down.

Moving Fluid Back Out of the Breast or Areola

Occasionally, no measures seem to help get a drop of milk flowing, and the breasts become rock hard. The ducts are full of milk, and the fluids that the breast uses to make milk are backed up around the ducts. This can lead to the entire breast becoming hard, including the areola. Once engorgement has reached this stage, the lymph passages may become blocked by the hardened breast tissue, further slowing the movement of fluid out of the breast.

Although at this point it may seem as if things couldn't possibly improve, it is possible to move the fluids back out of the breast and into the rest of the body. A skilled massage therapist can use lymphatic-drainage techniques to help the fluids flow, or you can use such a technique yourself.

To do this: Lie back on your bed with your head and a bit of your shoulder and arm dangling off the edge. Lift your arm up and out to expose your armpit. In this position, your whole breast moves upward and outward, which helps to open the lymphatic passages at the back of the breast. Very lightly, massage the breast with gentle strokes, moving first up toward the neck, then toward the shoulder, and finally toward the armpit. Use only the softest strokes, not deep pressure. The technique should not be painful. If it is, decrease the amount of pressure you are using. Massaging the breasts like this can rapidly relieve severe engorgement, especially when used with ice or cabbage and anti-inflammatory agents. (See "Cabbage, Herbs, and Anti-inflammatory Agents" later in this chapter.)

To soften a severely engorged areola enough to allow latching or pumping, try the useful technique known as "reverse pressure softening" originated by Jean Cotterman, a registered nurse and an International Board Certified Lactation Consultant. Start by gently placing your fingertips around all sides of the nipple, and apply gentle, sustained pressure to the areola for one minute. For very severe engorgement, hold the pressure for two or three minutes. You can sing a song or watch an egg timer to pass the time. The gentle pressure moves fluid away from the area. You may notice little dimples forming around the nipple and a softening of the areola. Once this happens, try latching the baby onto your breast or pumping some milk. Reverse pressure softening helps to make the areola more elastic, allowing the baby to latch more comfortably. The let-down then comes more quickly.

If engorgement is still so severe that the baby cannot get his chin in close enough for a good nursing position, try pressing under the areola for a few minutes to make a dip for the baby's chin. The fluid is moved away temporarily and doesn't immediately return. This technique can be repeated with each nursing session; it is even more effective as the breast softens. You can ask a lactation specialist for help with the technique. If you are severely engorged, it is best to call an expert anyway.

Sustained, severe engorgement is serious because it may damage the milk-producing capacity of the breast, at least for this baby. (It may still be possible to breastfeed other children later on.) For this reason, engorgement can quickly become a true lactation emergency. If this happens to you, it is best to see a breastfeeding expert as soon as possible. The best time to see one is during a weekday, as many consultants simply aren't available during evenings or on weekends. So, if things start getting bad on a Friday morning, don't wait for the crisis that will inevitably occur on Saturday. Instead, make an appointment to see an expert as soon as possible.

La Leche League Leaders are always available for phone calls, so don't hesitate to call one. A calm, reassuring voice over the phone has saved the day for many a nursing mother.

Cabbage, Herbs, and Anti-inflammatory Agents

Modern scientific studies have found cabbage leaves to be as effective as ice packs—no more, no less—in reducing engorgement. Many nursing mothers have found that cabbage leaves are more appealing than ice and really do relieve the swelling and discomfort of engorgement. Perhaps the shape of cabbage leaves originally suggested their use on the breasts, though it must be pointed out that cabbage has enjoyed hundreds of years of use for any sort of swelling. (Could their use for swelling have originated with a nursing woman?)

To prepare the cabbage, use the big leaves and cut the hard midrib out first. Then simply wrap the leaves around your breasts (inside your nursing bra so they stay in place). Replace the leaves once they have wilted. Some people claim that pounding the leaves soft before applying them to the breasts makes them more effective.

Another remedy for swelling is a poultice made of grated, raw potato or carrot. Carrots and potatoes have traditionally been used to reduce swelling of all sorts and are recommended by herbalists to ease the pain and discomfort of engorgement. Just be sure to wash the grated vegetables off of your breasts before nursing, so your baby doesn't taste or ingest them.

Some herbalists suggest poultices of wild violets to help with engorgement. You may be lucky enough to have violets growing in your yard, though dried violets may also be effective. Violets are rich in compounds that help swelling by stabilizing leaky capillaries. See the discussion on varicose veins in chapter 9 for other foods and herbs that may help to reduce swelling.

Many herbal books suggest that comfrey compresses on the breasts may relieve the soreness associated with engorgement. Comfrey is an excellent wound-healing plant; however, in my judgment, nursing mothers should avoid comfrey, especially comfrey root. Unless the product is certified toxin-free, it may contain significant amounts of toxic pyrrolizidine alkaloids. Certified toxin-free (less than one part per million, or <1 ppm, of pyrrolizidine alkaloids) comfrey leaf or root products are hard to find in the United States other than in tinctured form (see appendix C). This will hopefully change in the future, as comfrey is otherwise a very useful plant. If you do choose to use comfrey, I would recommend that you wash your breasts immediately afterwards and again before nursing. It is also wise to limit the time that the comfrey is in contact with your breasts, as engorged breasts may be particularly susceptible to absorbing plant constituents.

Internal use of comfrey is contraindicated during breastfeeding, and for very good reasons. The toxin causes irreversible and accumulative liver damage. Both adults and small children have developed liver failure as a result of consuming herbs high in toxic forms of pyrrolizidine alkaloids, but much smaller amounts may still cause liver damage—and without symptoms. Comfrey products are notoriously variable. A Canadian survey found that many comfrey products had high levels of the toxin; based on these findings, comfrey was banned in Canada. In Switzerland, the baby of a mother who had been using medicinal plants high in this toxin during her pregnancy and while breastfeeding developed fatal liver failure. While much of the damage to the baby probably occurred before birth, this incident could mean that breastfeeding babies are particularly susceptible to this toxin.

Although, in folk medicine, skin-irritating plants are sometimes applied to the breasts to provoke let-down, there are safer, more comfortable measures that can be used instead. Sometimes, pokeweed is recommended to relieve engorgement, perhaps due to its irritant properties. Be sure to read the discussion about pokeweed under "Mastitis" later in this chapter.

Sometimes, engorgement is the result of retaining a lot of water after birth. (Some lactation consultants suspect that large volumes of intravenous fluids given during and after delivery may worsen engorgement for some women.) Prescription diuretics have been used to help speed the removal of excess fluid from the body and thus the breasts, but herbal remedies may also work. An advantage of herbal diuretics is that they don't remove potassium from the body the way that prescription diuretics do. Herbalist Mechell Turner, IBCLC, has helped nursing mothers with diuretic herbs such as dandelion and corn silk. Many herbalists consider dandelion leaf to be the finest diuretic herb available. Note, though, that dandelion leaf may be a mild galactogogue. Interestingly, other species of this plant are used to increase milk in far-flung corners of the world—Tibet, Australia, and Europe, to name a few.

You may wish to use anti-inflammatory medications to relieve the pain of engorgement and reduce the irritation of breast tissue that comes with the buildup of fluids in the breast. In general, over-the-counter anti-inflammatory pain relievers (such as ibuprofen) are considered safe to use during breastfeeding, according to the American Academy of Pediatrics 2001 statement of drug use during lactation. Check with your doctor first to make sure that using anti-inflammatory medication is suitable and safe for your particular situation.

If you do not wish to use these medications, you could consider anti-inflammatory analgesic herbs such as willow bark instead. Willow bark contains salicin (a salicylate), and some healthcare providers may express concern that the use of this ingredient could lead to postpartum hemorrhage. However, according to herb scientists, unlike the synthetic salicylate aspirin, salicin does not thin the blood, cause stomach problems, provoke allergic reactions, or lead to Reye's syndrome. (Those who are allergic to aspirin may still wish to avoid salicin, however.) Salicin-containing herbs like willow bark are not thought to cause difficulties during breastfeeding.

Sore Nipples

Many mothers experience nipple pain or discomfort when their new baby latches on and starts to suck. Initial soreness is quite common, and it be can be downright painful. But once the milk starts flowing during the feeding, the soreness tends to diminish, and it should disappear by the time the nursing session is over. As the baby learns more about breastfeeding and the milk starts to flow more quickly after latching, soreness should become a thing of the past.

Some mothers have found that it can be a bit uncomfortable when their let-down takes awhile or when their baby vigorously works the breast in his eagerness to eat. But once the milk flows, the discomfort disappears, as do the baby's hunger pangs. In these situations, the nipples generally appear normal and aren't reddened or cracked. The initial discomfort decreases, and the nipples don't feel terribly sore between nursing sessions or become more painful with time.

Nipples that are sore, painful, or particularly tender between feedings, however, indicate that something isn't right. Most likely, the baby's nursing position and latch need to be checked. (See chapter 2 for a review of positioning and latching and for tips on finding breastfeeding helpers.) You may need the help of a lactation specialist who can show you how to improve the positioning and latch. Don't delay seeking help. Your nipple soreness may get much worse, making every breastfeeding session a painful ordeal. There are things you can do to help the situation, so take heart. Don't give up!

Soreness, Redness, Cracks, and Blisters

A baby that is well positioned at the breast, latches on correctly, and maintains a good latch throughout the nursing session creates very little friction on the tender areola or the nipple. When the baby's jaws are well back on the areola, the nipple lies close to the back of his throat, where it can come to no harm. The baby's tongue is extended out over his bottom gums, and he cups the breast from underneath. He creates gentle suction while he sucks and swallows, and this keeps the breast in place. If he is nursing properly, his mouth is applied well onto the areola, which puts a good amount of breast tissue between his jaws. When his jaws squeeze closed, milk is pushed into his mouth. He repeats this milking action until he has a good mouthful. Then he swallows and takes a breath.

However, it takes very little friction from the baby's mouth on the areola or nipple to quickly cause soreness. This soreness may progress to redness, cracks, and blisters around and on the nipple. It doesn't take very long for this to happen either, especially if the baby is able to nurse early and often. Even after just a few nursing sessions, your nipples may be cracked and sore. This is a definite sign that something is wrong. While this may occur on the first day or so of nursing, it can easily be overlooked in the hospital. Many times, mothers believe that nipple soreness is "normal" or a natural result of frequent nursing. Many do not tell the postpartum nurse about it, and not every nurse asks. Too often, mothers only realize that they have a latching problem after they return home and the pain and redness get really bad.

Don't wait to ask for help, no matter when sore nipples develop. In the early weeks, sore nipples are most likely due to poor positioning and latching. But some sore nipple conditions can occur later on, even months after birth. A breastfeeding specialist can sort out what is happening and make helpful suggestions. Once the underlying cause of the trauma is addressed, it may be only a matter of days before your nipples feel better. If they don't improve, then further help is needed. I have talked to many mothers who bore the pain and suffering of sore nipples for too long, hoping that things would improve. Two or three weeks into nursing, they were ready to quit (and who could blame them?). But, instead of giving up, they took action and called for the help they needed. They were able to continue breastfeeding after all.

There are many products on the market to help heal sore nipples, so ask a lactation specialist for guidance. Most of these products are for external use—creams and ointments, for example. Take a really hard look at the ingredients before using any of these creams. Nipples heal all by themselves, and very rapidly, once the cause of the trauma is fixed. If the latch has caused the problem, nipples can heal within just two or three days of correcting the latch—without having to put any creams or other products on them at all. Or simply gently rub some of your breast milk over your nipples after breastfeeding your baby.

Remember that any substance that is left on the nipples will be ingested by the baby as he nurses. In general, residues from water-based poultices, compresses, and herbal baths can be more easily removed from the breasts before nursing than those from creams and ointments. Nearly every nipple preparation has the potential to produce an allergic reaction in the mother or the baby. The one exception to this rule is hypoallergenic lanolin. Hypoallergenic lanolin is recommended by La Leche League and is widely available in drugstores. It may be a bit expensive, but a little goes a long way. Special processing has removed pesticides, as well as allergenic proteins. Lanolin not only speeds healing and prevents the formation of scabs, but also immediately soothes nipple pain. For maximum effectiveness, you need to apply small dabs frequently throughout the day and after nursing. Hypoallergenic lanolin is safe for use on the skin and won't harm your infant if he ingests some while nursing.

Creams containing comfrey aren't recommended, even though comfrey is a good wound healer and sore nipples are essentially open wounds. A comfrey poultice or tea wash isn't recommended either, due to comfrey's potentially toxic effects. See "Cabbage, Herbs, and Anti-Inflammatory Agents" in this chapter for a discussion of comfrey and its risks. There are other wound-healing herbs that are much safer for breastfeeding.

Likewise, using creams with vitamins A or D or putting vitamin E oil on the nipples may not be safe for your baby, who may easily ingest too much. Vitamin E can also cause dermatitis when externally applied, which would only add to your misery. Aloe vera gel isn't the best choice either, even though it is a superb wound healer. The gel not only tastes bitter to babies, but also contains small amounts of anthroquinones, constituents that can cause sensitive babies to develop cramps or diarrhea. If you do decide to use aloe vera gel, thoroughly remove it before every nursing session.

Tea rinses or poultices made with calendula (marigold), chamomile, and marshmallow are good options, as they have great skin-healing properties. (For information on making your own herbal tea, see chapter 7.) Ordinary black tea bags are sometimes used; you can make the tea and then cool the bags in the refrigerator before using them on your breasts. The tannins in black tea may speed healing, but they taste bitter; wash the tea off before nursing. Gentler wound-healing herbs like calendula are preferable.

While your nipples are healing, warm showers and gentle heat (warm packs or a not-too-hot water bottle) can be soothing and healing. Drying the nipples with blasts of hot air from a hair dryer is no longer recommended for sore nipples, as this only dehydrates and further irritates the skin.

Any time you have a persistent problem with sore nipples, get help from an expert. A lactation specialist may need to see you in person in order to watch you breastfeed, check the baby's positioning and latch, and look at your nipples. Nipples that are constantly sore even after the latch is fixed could indicate a bacterial infection or thrush. See your doctor if you have a rash or any unusual or persistent sores.

Bacterial Infection

If your nipples remain sore or the cracks refuse to heal despite a good latch, the cause of the problem may be bacterial. A bacterial infection can lead to the development of bacterial mastitis or even an abscess. If you suspect you have an infection, see your doctor. He or she may prescribe an appropriate antibiotic ointment or oral antibiotics.

Calendula (or marigold) flowers have been used as an anti-infective, skin-healing agent and may be the best herbal treatment for nipples infected with bacteria or thrush. (For more on thrush, see below.) Calendula can be applied as tea in a wet compress or as a poultice. A number of creams contain calendula. Be sure to read the other ingredients and ask yourself if these are good "first foods" for your baby. For very young babies, even the homeopathic creams should be removed before nursing.

Occasionally, an older baby who is already teething may accidentally bite while nursing. (Before you become too alarmed by the thought of being bitten while nursing, talk to a breastfeeding helper.) If you have a bite that doesn't heal quickly, a bacterial infection is likely to be present. I know one woman who used calendula cream to heal an old wound that had started with an accidental bite from her teething infant. She had tried various antibiotic creams for weeks, but nothing seemed to help. Then she discovered calendula, which helped heal the wound in a few days. Before rushing out to buy calendula, however, ask your breastfeeding helper if the herb is appropriate for your situation. This woman's child was already taking solid foods, so there was little risk from her use of the cream-based remedy on her nipples.

Whatever you do, there is a cardinal rule to follow if you suspect a bacterial infection: See your doctor as soon as possible. You don't want to risk a spread of the infection to the breast ducts, a problem known as mastitis, which is discussed later in this chapter.

Thrush

Thrush is such a large and complex topic that a full discussion of its causes and remedies is beyond the scope of this book. A brief overview of the topic follows. If you wish to learn more about thrush, see appendix A for a list of breastfeeding books that discuss it in more depth.

The fungus *Candida albicans* is thought to be the culprit that causes thrush. Candida is an organism that can live harmlessly on your skin and in your mucous membranes for many years without causing a problem. However, if something upsets the balance, candida can become invasive and start infecting the mucous membranes, causing inflammation and pain. What upsets this balance? Mothers with thrush frequently report that they, or their babies, had just finished a course of antibiotics. Fatigue from lack of sleep or a poor diet can also lead to thrush. Some mothers who are prone to vaginal yeast infections are prone to getting thrush, too.

Babies with thrush may develop spots in the mouth. These spots may be white and cheesy-looking, and may have reddened areas around them, but sometimes the baby's mouth can look entirely normal. Nursing mothers with thrush may notice that their nipples and areolae appear redder or pinker than usual or have a slightly pearly appearance. Thrush can also cause a burning sensation on the nipples, especially after nursing.

Without intervention, thrush can worsen, leading to pain deep in the breasts. There is no reliable lab test for thrush, as it is notoriously difficult to grow in a test tube. Other causes of nipple and breast pain need to be eliminated before diagnosing thrush. Fortunately, once diagnosed, thrush can be treated.

Thrush needs to be treated as quickly as possible. A fast and simple intervention is to wash the nipples with diluted vinegar (1 teaspoon of vinegar per cup of water) after breastfeeding. The acid in the vinegar discourages fungus. You can do this while waiting to see your doctor. The use of vinegar won't fight off an infection on its own, however—it just slows it down a little. Some mothers have found baking soda (1 teaspoon of baking soda dissolved in two cups water) to be helpful when applied as a wash, though this remedy is more often used with an eczema rash on the nipple.

You may also want to consider a course of immune-boosting herbs such as echinacea to help rally your body's defenses. According to herb expert James Duke in his book *The Green Pharmacy,* the best antifungal herbs are echinacea—for its immune-boosting effects—and garlic—for its many antifungal compounds. (Other compounds in garlic help fight off bacterial infection as well.) Some babies find garlic-laced breast milk difficult to digest, while others nurse all the more because they seem to like the taste.

Echinacea can immediately boost your immune system by making infection-fighting cells more active. It is rarely allergenic, but if you have a disease that affects your immune system, be sure to consult with a healthcare provider before self-treating with this herb. Possible side effects on the breastfeeding baby have yet to be identified. You can take echinacea in capsules, as a tea, or from a tincture; dried, pressed juice tablets are probably the most effective form, though tinctures can also be effective. The tea or tincture may taste truly awful to you, but it should make your mouth feel tingly and numb if it is a good preparation.

Dr. Jack Newman, a pediatrician who specializes in caring for breastfeeding women and children, suggests that a short course of gentian violet will soon tell you whether you're dealing with thrush. A full description of how to use gentian violet to treat thrush is available at www.breastfeedingonline.com/newman.html and in Dr. Newman's book *The Ultimate Breastfeeding Book of Answers* (see appendix A). Gentian violet has the same beautiful purple color of gentian flowers, but it is a synthetic chemical that has been used to treat infected wounds for over a century. Seek expert guidance before trying gentian violet. It is available over the counter, but preparations of it need to be properly diluted. Gentian violet should be used for no more than a week at a time.

Herpes Lesions on the Breast

Nursing with a herpes lesion on or near the areola is potentially fatal for a newborn. If you have a history of herpes, see your doctor immediately if a lesion appears on your breast, especially in the early days of breastfeeding. Typically, a baby can nurse if the lesion is covered, or if he exclusively nurses from the other breast. Call on your breastfeeding helpers for more information on your options.

There are other herbal remedies for thrush you might try as well. Dr. Newman and another well-known pediatrician, Dr. Jay Gordon, have found grapefruit seed extract (GSE) to be useful in treating thrush (not *grapeseed* extract, but *grapefruit seed* extract). Dr. Gordon recommends that the liquid extract should first be tried on the nipples *after* nursing. (The extract is bitter, so your baby won't like the taste.) Dr. Gordon has found that using GSE externally works more quickly than using it internally. You can read more about his approach on his web site: www.drjaygordon.com. Alternatively, Dr. Newman suggests that nursing mothers first try GSE internally, then, if that approach fails, try applying it externally. This approach may be preferable with a very young or allergy-prone baby. GSE itself is nontoxic, but some brands contain synthetic antiseptics that should be avoided.

Other topical antifungal herbal treatments include black walnut and tea tree oils, but both have drawbacks. Black walnut is a very bitter herb, and your baby may resist nursing when you use it topically. Tea tree oil can be toxic when taken internally, so I question whether it is wise to apply it externally to the nipples. There is a risk that the baby would ingest some amount every time he nurses, and toddlers have been poisoned after consuming very small amounts of tea tree oil. In addition, the strong smell of tea tree oil on the breast may trigger breathing difficulties in a newborn. English herbalist David Hoffmann says that calendula is an effective antifungal, whether used internally or externally. This is a safer alternative to tea tree oil.

If you have chronic yeast infections and have been told to change your diet to exclude all sugars and yeast products, doing so will not decrease the lactose sugar in your breast milk, which is what the breast thrush is thriving on. But avoiding sugars and yeast products may improve your digestion overall, which, in turn, may improve your ability to fight off a yeast infection throughout your body, including your breasts. Fixing an inflammatory condition in your gut can help overall body functioning. Focusing on a good diet is a solid foundation from which to fight any chronic, opportunistic infection.

Lactobacillus bacteria, taken either in yogurt or capsule form, can do wonders for restoring gastrointestinal health and is recommended by even the most conservative nutritionists, especially if you're taking antibiotics. It is sometimes suggested that rubbing the powdered lactobacillus bacteria (from capsules) on baby's gums will help. Keep in mind, however, that the exclusively breastfed baby will already have almost nothing but *Lactobacillus bifidus* bacteria in his mouth and GI tract, so why add more in the form of an expensive supplement?

Giving cow protein, in yogurt or probiotic supplements, to babies under the age of six months is a significant allergenic risk, because cow's milk protein is a prime allergen. It is much safer to wait until six months of age, when your child is ready to eat solid foods. Some babies are extraordinarily sensitive to cow's milk protein and will react to even the denatured protein found in yogurt.

Author and herbal expert James Duke loves to develop ways to get his medicine in food. He could publish a whole cookbook of the recipes he has written for specific medicinal purposes. In his book *The Green Pharmacy,* he shares his "Candicidal Soup" recipe, which exploits the medicinal quantities of onion and garlic—think French onion soup. To this base he adds flavor with thrush-fighting sage, thyme, cloves, and black pepper. Nursing mothers may want to go easy on thyme and skip the sage (taken daily, sage may lower your milk supply). He also adds a big dollop of yogurt to each bowl.

Preparing the soup in large quantities and eating it frequently can help fight an existing yeast infection or prevent the occurrence of an infection when antibiotics are used. Adding garlic and onions to your daily diet will also help wear down the "yeasty beasties" and keep their behavior within bounds.

Antifungal prescription medications such as fluconazole may be needed when simpler treatments fail. Unlike vaginal yeast infections, which can be treated with a single dose, breast yeast infections may require a considerably longer course of treatment with fluconazole or similar medicines. Talk to your healthcare provider about whether this option is appropriate for your situation.

Other Reasons for Nipple Soreness

Even if your baby has been nursing for quite a while, his latch may change if you introduce a bottle or a pacifier. This can lead to unexpected nipple soreness. It's also possible that your nipples will become sore once your baby starts eating solid foods, usually as a result of contact dermatitis and the rash that comes with it. Rinse your nipples after nursing or give your child water to drink after eating. This will rinse away any food particles that could irritate the skin.

Occasionally, rashes and sores on the nipples can signal a serious health condition. When in doubt, consult with your breastfeeding helpers and your doctor. No matter what your circumstances, if you have a skin condition on your breasts that doesn't clear up after the usual treatments, seek the help of a knowledgeable dermatologist who can work with a lactation specialist. You may need to specifically request such a consultation. Getting a diagnosis from a dermatologist will help you decide what treatment choices are right for you.

Plugged Ducts, Mastitis, and Other Painful Conditions

The issue of breast pain is surprisingly complex, as there are many possible causes. Sometimes, a number of factors may jointly create a problem. Other times, a simple breast condition may worsen into a more serious condition. To figure out why you're having breast pain, seek the help of someone who is knowledgeable about this topic and can take the time to thoroughly discuss your particular situation. Pain is a signal that things aren't right. It demands your attention and the attention of your healthcare providers as well.

A lactation specialist can help you figure out the cause of the pain and offer suggestions on what has worked well for other mothers in your situation. These days, painful breast conditions can be helped. Immediate weaning is not the answer. In fact, your problem may not even require an interruption in breastfeeding. You can continue nursing while finding solutions that work for you.

Plugged Ducts and Other Painful Lumps and Bumps in the Breast

Many nursing mothers experience plugged ducts. A plugged duct is just what it sounds like: a blocked duct that prevents the milk from flowing. The duct is blocked by precipitated milk. (The milk is thick and sometimes granular in texture.) Signs of a plugged duct include a tender spot, a slightly reddish area, or a sore lump. Often, plugged ducts make their presence known gradually. Sometimes they even change locations. Some plugs occur deep within the breast tissue, while others seem to end up in the areola where you can see them under the skin as a white bump. A plugged duct at the areola can make breastfeeding somewhat painful because the baby's mouth puts pressure on the duct when nursing.

Generally, a plugged duct causes mild to moderate localized pain. You may feel okay otherwise, though some mothers run a low-grade fever (less than 101° F). You may notice that a small section of the breast behind the plug becomes hard as the milk cakes, or backs up in the duct. Usually, the skin won't become hot, though.

Plugged ducts often appear after a baby first starts sleeping through the night or when the mother goes back to work and isn't nursing as often as before. In other words, the ducts get plugged when the regular pattern of milk removal is changed.

Ultrasound Treatment

Dr. Jack Newman says that if a blocked duct has not cleared within forty-eight hours (which is unusual), therapeutic ultrasound often works. Ultrasound treatment can be arranged at a local physiotherapy office or sports medicine clinic. Many ultrasound therapists aren't yet aware of this use of ultrasound. Talk to your doctor or healthcare provider about this option.

Some mothers are particularly susceptible to plugged ducts. Mothers who have an oversupply of milk, for example, are prone to developing plugs, perhaps because their breastfeeding babies can't regularly drink all of the milk that is present in the breast. This can lead to repeated engorgement, and then to plugged ducts. Sometimes, a poor latch causes poor drainage from the breast, which results in the formation of a plug. Once a plug slows or stops the flow of milk from a section of the breast, the surrounding tissues may become engorged, which can cause inflammation in the breast, or mastitis. You can read about mastitis later in this chapter.

Plugged ducts can also result from wearing a bra that's too tight, using an under-wire support bra, or wearing a bra to bed—all of which can slow drainage from some parts of the breast. Wear more loosely fitting clothing if you think a plug has developed. Sometimes, a plug forms right at the nipple. (You may see a white spot there.) You can sometimes soak off the milk secretions using warm, wet compresses. If you seem to be prone to plugged ducts, talk to a La Leche League Leader or other lactation specialist to determine your particular risk factors.

There are many ways to treat a plugged duct. First and foremost, you have to get your milk flowing and keep it flowing. Nurse your baby frequently and make sure he is latched on well enough to thoroughly drain the breast. Your baby may become fussy if the plug slows down the milk flow, so be prepared. Avoid lengthy periods between nursing sessions. If necessary, set your alarm clock to wake yourself during the night for feedings. Sleep is important, but unplugging the duct is even more important, because you don't want to develop mastitis.

As you breastfeed, point your baby's chin in the direction of the plug, which may help move the plug downward, encouraging the flow of fluids. Try different nursing positions to see if a particular one seems to bring relief. You can also nurse on your hands and knees so that your breasts hang down, letting gravity help the plug to break up. While nursing, knead the plugged breast gently. Breast massage and breast compression may help to dislodge plugs and get the milk flowing again. Dr. Jack Newman believes that breast compression can help prevent plugs from

What Is a Galactocele?

Some women find that a plug causes the duct behind it to expand into what is called a galactocele, or a milk-filled cavity. A galactocele doesn't usually hurt because it remains somewhat soft, but it can grow to the size of a golf ball. These lumps are filled with milk or a cheeselike substance, which helps to distinguish them from other breast lumps. The contents of the galactocele can be drawn out using a needle, but the galactocele often forms again soon afterwards.

There aren't many known remedies for healing galactoceles. One mother I know found that gently slowing her milk production, using the antigalactogogue herb white sage, helped to shrink a large galactocele and prevented it from recurring. White sage was a familiar friend to her, being Native American, yet she still sought herbalist assistance before using it. Note that temporarily slowing milk production with herbs is a traditional approach in many societies whenever mothers experience certain breast problems. However, antigalactogogue herbs must be used minimally, carefully, and with expert help to prevent a too-large drop in milk supply. Read more about these herbs in chapter 7.

recurring if used at the first sign of difficulty. You can read about breast compression in chapter 7 and about breast massage in chapters 5 and 7.

If the plugs are deep in the breast tissue, a warm massage bath may help. Add soothing herbs such as marshmallow root, oats, or fenugreek to warm water—enough to make the bath slippery. The slippery mixture will reduce friction on the skin while helping your hands slide gently over your breasts. Always massage the breasts gently. Irritated, inflamed tissues need special care to avoid being damaged.

Dry or moist heat over the plugged area can ease the discomfort and fight off infection. Try warm showers, heating pads, hot water bottles, or warm, wet compresses. Just make sure the water doesn't get too hot. Last but not least, get your rest. While there doesn't seem to be much time for sleep when you have a new baby, breast problems are often a warning that you need to take things more slowly. Think of rest as the "medicine" that can help you fight off infection.

Some mothers who suffer from chronic plugs and mastitis have found relief by adding a rich source of choline to their diet. Dietary choline is found in the form of lecithin, a waxy, oily substance that occurs naturally in plants and animals. Soybeans contain significant amounts of lecithin. You can buy lecithin in the form of capsules or granules in health-food stores. (Read more about choline in chapter 6.)

To prevent plugged ducts, lactation expert Dr. Ruth Lawrence recommends taking 1 tablespoon of liquid or granulated lecithin daily. Or take 1 lecithin capsule (1200 mg) 3–4 times per day. It may also be helpful to reduce the amount of saturated fats you consume (try avoiding trans-fats completely), while increasing your consumption of unsaturated fats, such as olive oil and those ever-important omega-3 fatty acids (see chapter 6).

Once in a while, what a nursing mother thinks is a plugged duct may actually be a supernumerary, or extra, breast. A supernumerary breast usually looks like nothing more than a wart and is often located in the upper part of the breast near the armpit. After birth, the area can become engorged, sometimes swelling to the size of a tennis ball. Because supernumerary breasts may not have ducts that connect to the true breast, or even an opening to the surface of the skin, they can become hard and uncomfortable after the birth. Cabbage leaves applied to the area may help. (See "Cabbage, Herbs, and Anti-inflammatory Agents" earlier in this chapter.) Supernumerary breasts typically disappear on their own, since milk isn't being removed from them, but they will return with the next birth. Ask a lactation specialist for more information about them. They are not as rare as you might imagine.

Mastitis

The term "mastitis" means inflammation of the breast. Mastitis is painful and may produce flu-like symptoms, including a fever. When you have mastitis, you may feel achy and out of sorts. You may have a lump or a plugged duct. (See the preceding section on plugged ducts.) One breast may appear red and swollen and feel hot, while the other breast may appear normal. If both breasts are affected, your baby is just a few weeks old, or you have a fever over 101° F, call your doctor immediately. You may have acquired an infection at the hospital and need immediate medical attention.

Breast inflammation isn't necessarily a breast infection. Any time milk is stopped from flowing, fluid buildup causes inflammation. A low-grade fever, body aches, and breast pain soon follow. Emptying the breast frequently will help reduce the inflammation, whatever its cause. You can continue to breastfeed with mastitis. Sudden weaning isn't necessary and can actually worsen the pain and inflammation.

Mastitis seems to go hand-in-hand with feeling discouraged and overwhelmed. Some mothers have found that when they take on too much they suffer a bout of mastitis. If you have developed mastitis, the best thing to do is go to bed and nurse your baby frequently. Moist or dry heat and gentle massage on the swollen spots also helps. (See the remedies for plugged ducts described earlier in this chapter.)

Maximizing your rest, getting some much needed sleep, and keeping the affected breast empty can often prevent a bacterial infection from developing. However, if you don't feel much better by the next day or if you have the signs and symptoms of a bacterial infection (high fever, intense breast pain), see your doctor for a diagnosis. Bacterial infections must be appropriately and effectively treated to prevent complications. Antibiotics may be needed.

Unlike a plugged duct, bacterial mastitis comes on suddenly. A hot, red area, painful to the touch, often develops on the breast. A fever over 101° F and flu-like symptoms are common. You may have red streaks from the infection site or notice pus or blood in your milk.

Bacterial mastitis can be caused by a number of things. Stress and fatigue can weaken the immune system, inviting an infection. A first bout of bacterial mastitis often comes just a few weeks after birth, which is a stressful time even if breastfeeding is going well. Some mothers develop mastitis soon after returning to work. Dealing with a family crisis, or even a happy family get-together, can precipitate infection. If the rest of the family gets a cold, "Nurse Mom" may end up with bacterial mastitis. Mothers with anemia or diabetes are very susceptible to infection, too. Another cause is cracks on the nipple that allow skin bacteria such as staph or strep to invade breast tissue.

If a bacterial infection is diagnosed, appropriate antibiotics will clear it up quickly and prevent abscesses. (Abscesses are essentially boils, or walled-off pockets of pus deep in the tissues—our body's imperfect way of protecting healthy tissue. Abscesses often require surgical incision and drainage. Seek a surgeon who knows how to treat abscess in a breastfeeding-friendly way.) Prescribed antibiotics should be effective against staph *(Staphylococcus aureus)*—the most common bacteria associated with mastitis and abscess. Penicillinase-resistant penicillins or cephalosporins are currently preferred for treating mastitis. You do not need to stop breastfeeding your baby to use them.

A number of herbal remedies are traditionally used to treat mastitis. But because you may suffer serious consequences from ineffective treatment, and the herbals have not been proven effective when used alone, these remedies should be used only as a complement to antibiotics, and not in place of antibiotics. Many mothers have found herbal remedies to be very helpful in the early stages of mastitis, when used with the basic interventions of rest and frequent nursing sessions. The remedies can be started immediately upon first feeling ill, but if you are not feeling better after twenty-four hours, medical attention should be sought. If antibiotics become necessary, there is no reason to stop using the herbs. Herbs and antibiotics can work together to overcome the infection.

Immune-system-stimulating herbs such as echinacea, adaptogenic or tonic herbs such as ginseng, and vitamin C are often recommended for treating mastitis. Other herbal remedies, however, are more controversial, perhaps none more so than pokeweed, or poke. Pokeweed is traditionally used to treat breast infections and is also thought to encourage lymphatic drainage. While homeopathic preparations of poke may be effective and safe, herbal material preparations are another story. Fresh poke plants can be extremely irritating to sensitive skin. Using the fresh plant as a poultice could cause problems. Using pokeweed preparations internally can also be dangerous, depending on what stage of its growth cycle the plant was harvested. Poke is eaten as a food in the southern United States, where people know how to go about it. Nevertheless, it has still caused occasional mass poisonings. Because pokeweed is potentially toxic, an herbalist must have considerable skill to prepare a safe product. In addition, it's easy to take too much; poke is a powerful herb that demands respect. Do not use it on your own unless you are very, very familiar with the plant. Most of us should avoid herbal preparations made from pokeweed and stick to nontoxic homeopathic versions.

Vasospasm

Mothers who suffer pain while nursing sometimes notice that their nipples blanch, or turn white, right after the baby comes off the breast. Some mothers have also noticed that their nipples blanch whenever they step out of the shower or when they take their bras off. The nipples turn white because the blood vessels go into spasm, or squeeze shut (a "vasospasm"). When the blood vessels eventually open again and the blood flows back, the nipples can turn quite red. Vasospasm can cause burning pain in the nipple and breast, very similar to the pain associated with thrush. However, this pain will not respond to the treatments used for thrush.

Vasospasm often occurs if the baby is compressing the nipple. If this is happening, the nipple may look misshapen when it comes out of the baby's mouth. Vasospasm also can occur with nipple infections (thrush or bacterial), strong let-down reflex, or an oversupply of milk. Women with a family history of Raynaud's phenomenon (where the fingers go into vasospasm when exposed to cold) are at a higher risk of developing vasospasm of the nipple. If you suspect you may be suffering from this problem, talk to a lactation specialist. See your doctor if pain persists after any breastfeeding issues are solved.

Vasospasm can be successfully treated with the prescription drug nifedipine. Adding calcium and magnesium supplements to the diet has long been used to treat nipple vasospasm, too. A suggested dose is 1000 mg of calcium with 500 mg of magnesium per day. (Interestingly, some lactation consultants report that taking 1000 mg of liquid calcium per day can help with oversupply of milk as well.) If you are having vasospasms, it is wise to avoid sudden temperature changes, caffeine, and tobacco. Warming the nipples quickly after nursing helps blood return to them, which reduces the pain.

Standardized extract of ginkgo leaf is a common herbal therapy for Raynaud's phenomenon. Because ginkgo improves blood flow in peripheral capillaries, it may help with nipple vasospasm as well. Some people should not use ginkgo if they need to use certain drugs such as coumadin or aspirin, are planning to have surgery, or have certain blood clotting disorders. There are no known reports of adverse effects in infants whose mothers use ginkgo while breastfeeding, though some women report a mild increase in milk flow after let-down.

Fibrocystic Breast Disease

Mastalgia is a condition in which breast tissue becomes painful and lumpy before a menstrual period. The condition may occur or recur when menstrual periods return after postpartum. Some women have found that evening primrose oil (EPO), which is rich in certain types of essential fatty acids, can help alleviate lumpy breasts. EPO may work for nursing mothers, and there are no known adverse effects with its use while nursing.

Other herbs can also be helpful for treating mastalgia, particularly chasteberry, which is a well-known remedy approved for use in Germany. However, chasteberry may reduce your milk supply when taken for prolonged periods and in the dose range usually suggested for mastalgia. For more about chasteberry, see chapter 11.

🌿 🌿 🌿

There are many conditions that can result in nipple or breast pain. A lactation specialist can help you sort out the likely villains or identify those factors that may be contributing to the problem. Finding the actual cause of breast or nipple problems sometimes requires a visit to the doctor. It's important to seek medical assistance if you have persistent, unusual, or severe symptoms. If at first no cause can be found for persistent breast problems, please continue to seek help. If one provider isn't helpful, keep on looking. A La Leche League Leader can call on that organization's medical advisors if this is what you need. Persist in finding helpers who respect your breastfeeding efforts and who will support you in whatever you decide to do, even if no explanation for the breast pain can be found. (This is rarely the case, but it can happen.) Whether you continue breastfeeding or not, finding someone who will listen to you and respect your feelings is important for both you and your baby.

*W*hen You Have a Health Problem

At some point, you may become ill or experience a health problem that requires treatment.* This chapter is about what to do in the event of an illness and how to keep yourself healthy. Just to reassure you: It's perfectly safe for you to breastfeed even if you become ill. Breastfeeding is healthy for both you and your baby, and there are very few medical situations that would require you to stop nursing your child, even temporarily. If your healthcare provider suggests that you wean your baby so that you can receive medical treatment, seek a second opinion. Talk to a lactation specialist who understands your situation and can help you find ways to continue nursing. Share the information your lactation specialist gives you with your doctor so that, together, the two of you can develop a treatment plan that, if at all possible, will not interfere with your breastfeeding.

---

*This chapter deals with general health issues. For information specifically on breast problems, see chapter 8. For information on milk supply problems, see chapter 7. For information on problems with your baby's health, see chapter 10.

Many nursing mothers mistakenly believe that during an illness, they have no choice but to suffer through the symptoms. Yet, there are many options for relieving symptoms—including prescription drugs, over-the-counter medications, and herbal remedies—that are quite compatible with breastfeeding. If you're dealing with a serious or persistent illness, it's best to see a doctor first to discuss your symptoms, get a medical diagnosis, and choose appropriate treatment.

For a review of using herbs and medications safely while breastfeeding, see chapter 4. Appendix C contains safety ratings of specific herbs you may wish to take.

Common Illnesses and Health Problems

This chapter addresses questions about common illnesses and health problems frequently asked by nursing mothers. Sometimes, nursing mothers want to use a certain remedy but are told, or read somewhere, that the remedy should be avoided during breastfeeding. Naturally, nursing mothers want to be sure that an herbal product that has been recommended to them is nontoxic and not expected to cause problems during breastfeeding. On the following pages, you will find information about some common herbal treatment options. This information isn't intended as a substitute for medical treatment. You should always see a healthcare professional who can diagnose your illness and suggest possible treatments.

Infections

For serious infections, always consult with a physician who can determine what type of infection you have and what conventional medications are commonly used to treat it. The consequences of not treating an infection can be serious. Antibiotics are a first line of defense, and the vast majority of them can be used while breastfeeding. Natural treatments are fine in addition to an antibiotic and may very well speed your recovery. But when it comes to infections, natural remedies are not always a safe substitute for conventional treatment. Severe or persistent symptoms indicate the need for antibiotics. In such cases, a lot is riding on the outcome, and it may be best for your health—and therefore your baby's health—to accept antibiotic treatment.

Occasionally, breastfeeding babies may develop diarrhea when their mothers are taking antibiotics. This is a possible sign of a sensitivity or an allergy to the medication. Talk with your doctor about other antibiotics that will fight your infection, and then change the prescription as needed.

When taking any antibiotics, it's helpful to maintain your gastrointestinal health. A course of antibiotics can kill off not only the infection but also the good bacteria in your system, giving other unpleasant organisms the chance to multiply and create an opportunistic infection. Thrush, a fungal infection, is a well-known example. Nursing mothers who use antibiotics may end up getting breast thrush. (Read more about thrush in chapter 8.) A good preventive measure is to take probiotics: eat yogurt, drink kefir (a yogurt beverage), or take probiotic capsules (a nonherbal dietary supplement), all of which can prevent thrush overgrowths in the gastrointestinal tract and seem to inhibit thrush infections in the vagina and breasts as well. Look for probiotics in the refrigerated section of health-food stores. All of these products contain "good guy" bacteria (acidophilus species and others), which will maintain or even restore the natural mix of bacteria in the gut. Adding a daily dose of fresh or powdered garlic is helpful, too, if your baby isn't bothered by onions and garlic. (Most babies like the taste, but a few become fussy.) Garlic contains natural thrush-fighting components that are absorbed into the bloodstream and make their way to the breasts.

For bothersome viral infections like colds or the flu, antibiotics don't help. They haven't been proven to shorten the duration of either illness, so there is good reason to avoid their use. Over-the-counter medications can relieve your symptoms, but keep in mind that medications containing antihistamines or pseudoephedrine may have the unintended effect of lowering your milk supply. (Antihistamines and pseudoephedrine are common ingredients in allergy and cold medicines.) Ask a pharmacist for help in avoiding these ingredients.

A number of herbs are generally safer alternatives to over-the-counter medications for cold and flu, and their anti-inflammatory effects will help you feel better faster. Talk to an herbal practitioner to get help in choosing herbs that may be worth trying. Herbal books suggest numerous herbal remedies that may comfort you during a cold or a bout with the flu and may even help fight off minor infections. However, be aware that some of these herbs may affect your milk supply—in particular, sage, thyme, and parsley. Although inhaling the soothing and infection-fighting aroma of thyme in a steam bath won't affect your milk supply, some nursing mothers have reported that using cough lozenges made with sage seemed to lower their supply. See chapter 7 for more information about herbs and milk supply.

Immune-strengthening herbs can be used to stimulate your immune system to help fight off an infection. Some of the herbs that may be helpful include elderberry, garlic, and onion—all of which have been used by nursing mothers without any controversial effects. Echinacea is the most commonly used herb for strengthening the immune system; evidence suggests this herb may prevent a cold if taken when symptoms start and may shorten the duration of the cold. Products vary in quality, and not all work well. Echinacea isn't known to have harmful effects during breastfeeding, so it should be a safe choice for you. However, if you have allergies or an immune-related disease, it's best to investigate the herb more thoroughly before use.

Another herb, goldenseal, has a long history of use in fighting a wide range of infections and illnesses, including dysentery, cholera, and giardiasis. Its anti-infective activity is due mainly to berberine and related compounds, also found in the herbs barberry and Oregon grape. Berberine-containing herbs have been found to be effective against infections in the mouth, throat, and gastrointestinal tract, as well as infections of the skin or mucous membranes. Berberine not only has a germ-killing action but also helps to stabilize the mucous membranes it comes in contact with, thus drying up the nose or stopping diarrhea. Because berberine is barely absorbed from the GI tract, goldenseal and similar herbs do not work for infections of the blood or the breast.

Some herbalists have suggested that goldenseal, as a "drying herb," may lower milk supply, but I don't know of any cases where this has happened to a nursing mother. Plants containing berberine alkaloids should be avoided in pregnancy. It is best to use a small dose at a time and to limit the duration of use to three days at a time. Consult an herbalist before using larger doses.

Vitamin C, an important antioxidant, is widely recommended for fighting infection and relieving inflammation. To get more vitamin C, concentrate on eating citrus fruits, taking rose hips in pills, or consuming other rich sources of vitamin C. Supplementing your diet with vitamin C will not increase its content in your breast milk. For acute infections, doses of several grams of vitamin C per day are often recommended. However, suddenly starting such large doses may give you diarrhea, so you may want to use a smaller dose or look for sustained-release forms of vitamin C instead. When breastfeeding, always think moderation.

A Note about Berberine

Berberine alkaloids, especially hydrastine, can have toxic effects when injected into laboratory animals, prompting some to warn against their use during breastfeeding. However, berberine, like many other saponins, probably doesn't enter breast milk in significant amounts because it is barely absorbed from the GI tract.

It is worth noting that goldenseal is a plant that is considered threatened in its natural habitat and shouldn't be used for this reason. (Alternatives such as barberry or Oregon grape are preferable.) However, if a manufacturer uses cultivated goldenseal, this product would be a good alternative. Appendix B includes contact information for United Plant Savers, which was founded to protect endangered

Hay Fever, Allergies, and Asthma

Hay fever and other environmental allergies can be miserable to endure. Antihistamines are the usual treatment, but they may lower milk supply and therefore aren't the best choice for nursing mothers. A good herbal book will list many herbs considered useful for hay fever and allergies.

Alternative remedies for nasal allergies include freeze-dried nettle, kudzu, and passionflower. Nettle and kudzu have both been used as galactogogues (meaning they increase milk), though only nettle is well known for this. Freeze-dried nettle can be very helpful with a runny nose, but its ability to increase milk may be an unwanted effect for some nursing mothers. (See chapter 7 for more on milk supply issues.) Other forms of nettle may also be helpful, but the freeze-dried products are the ones for which there is some evidence of efficacy.

Passionflower (specifically, *Passiflora incarnata*) is most typically used as a mild nervine, or nerve tonic, to help with sleep. Passionflower can contain very small amounts of harmine and harmaline alkaloids. The amount varies depending on how the plant was grown and harvested. The German Commission E specifies that passionflower products must contain less than 0.01 percent of harmine alkaloids. Look for products that follow this rule.

It is not at all clear what, if any, potential effect passionflower may have on milk supply, though there is evidence that some effect is possible. Passionflower has been used for weaning, which would suggest it aids in diminishing milk supply. But two other species of *Passiflora*, as well as other plants that contain harmine alkaloids, are traditionally used as galactogogues and therefore increase milk. The alkaloids are also known to be uterotonic (meaning they cause uterine contractions), so be aware of this effect. At this time, I know of no lactation-related adverse effects attributed to the use of passionflower.

Note: Other species of passionflower contain potentially toxic compounds and should be avoided. The species used in herbal products—*Passiflora incarnata*—does not. But be sure to choose a product made by a reputable company. There is also a homeopathic form that is safe for use. If you plan to use passionflower for allergies, keep its use occasional and do not take it for extended periods of time without first consulting an herbalist.

Many sufferers of hay fever have found that changing their diet can greatly relieve their symptoms. You may want to try to find out which foods, if any, you may be sensitive to; the usual allergenic culprits are often found through a period of trial and error. Eliminating dairy, wheat, eggs, or beef products has helped many people overcome the annual return of their runny nose and itchy eyes. Hunting down food allergens takes time and self-denial of what are often favorite foods. You have to be prepared for a disciplined approach to food for quite a few weeks. It may take more than a couple months to see the full benefits of these efforts.

Fatigue

Caring for a baby or toddler is tiring. Lack of sleep can bring on a numbness of mind and body that makes even getting dressed in the morning a monumental chore. A poor diet may also contribute to the rapid onset of fatigue. Try adding plenty of natural sources of iron and B-vitamins to your diet to maintain your energy level. Sometimes, all you really need is a nice long nap and a solid night's sleep.

Persistent fatigue may be the result of more than lack of sleep. If your fatigue isn't relieved by rest and a decent diet, be sure to see a doctor. You may be suffering from anemia, a thyroid condition, or depression. Whatever the cause of your fatigue may be, it is important to seek solutions.

If anemia is the source of your fatigue, raising your iron levels will help. You may need more than your prenatal vitamins after birth. But taking an additional iron supplement may make you constipated and cause your breastfeeding baby to become fussy. Iron-rich foods and herbs may be a lot easier on both you and your baby.

Following are some helpful tips for increasing iron:

- Try blackstrap molasses: This is not the light cooking molasses often used for gingerbread; this stuff is black and thick and contains 20 to 40 percent of the daily requirement for iron in a mere tablespoon. It is a bit strong and bitter, but you may acquire a taste for it. Check the label for iron content, as many brands have been partially refined and contain less iron. Blackstrap molasses is rich in a whole range of minerals, particularly sulfur.

- Add dried fruits such as raisins, apricots, prunes, cherries, and figs—especially black mission figs—to your diet.

- Add iron simply by using cast-iron cooking pots and pans.

What about Detoxification and "Heroic" Bowel Programs?

Traditional healing practices around the world share a certain emphasis on the digestive tract as a way to fix many other seemingly unrelated problems in the body. So, treatment of a wide number of difficulties, from indigestion to fatigue, may start with improving bowel health.

Hand-in-hand with this approach comes a secondary focus on improving the function of the liver and gall bladder. For example, herbs called "bitters" are used to stimulate appetite and improve digestive function. Many bitters have been shown to increase bile flow (cholagogues) and other digestive juices, thereby improving digestion and nutrient absorption in the gastrointestinal tract.

Herbalist traditions prescribe various other remedies that may also soothe the lining of the GI tract or act as nonstimulating bulk laxatives. Indeed, research and common sense suggest that the GI tract isn't endlessly forgiving of all foods that we eat. Malabsorption and inflammatory states do exist in the bowel, and they may cause or worsen a wide array of illnesses, as well as more general states of malaise, fatigue, and exhaustion.

Many so-called detoxification programs use herbs that are known to improve liver function: milk thistle, licorice, or schisandra, for example. Sometimes, however, herbalists warn against "detoxifying" while breastfeeding, fearing that these herbs will suddenly dump "toxins" into the bloodstream. This is a basic misunderstanding of how these herbs work. Herbs such as milk thistle and wu wei zi (schisandra) have been shown to improve the liver cells' ability to function, including their ability to metabolize toxins and eliminate them from the body through bile and the GI tract. They can even restore the liver's ability to function by regenerating new liver tissue, as well as fend off additional damage to the liver. These herbs help the liver work better at removing any circulating toxins; this is good for the breastfeeding baby, as removing the toxins from his mother's bloodstream also removes them from the breast milk.

Heroic bowel programs are another method of purging body toxins. In the old days of conventional medicine, massive or "heroic" amounts of purgative herbs were used to treat patients. Methods for purging patients of "toxins" were used by the early naturopaths and country doctors, too. The approach is still advocated by some herbalist traditions that emphasize "cleaning out the bowels." These traditions hold that the bowels are full of what is variously described as old, dried feces, mucus, or other "toxic" material. Invariably, their rapid and dramatic removal solves the problem.

Such "heroic remedies," as herbalist Susun Weed has called them, have an obvious effect on the body, which may impress the patient as being "strong medicine." Given that many of these programs employ powerful purgative herbs that can cause cramps and diarrhea in nursing mothers, they are quite capable of causing cramps and diarrhea in breastfeeding babies as well. Nursing mothers who have frequent, loose stools may become dehydrated and lose vital minerals. In many traditions, including traditional European and Chinese herbalism, purgative herbs are considered harmful for the mother-baby pair. I generally recommend avoiding such remedies while breastfeeding.

- Choose anemia-fighting herbs such as nettle and watercress (both are also mild galactogogues), rose hips, yellow dock root, and burdock root. All of these herbs are typically used to relieve postpartum anemia. Parsley may also be used, but, if taken in large doses, it can lower milk supply.

There are a number of excellent herbal products available to build iron supply. Often, these products use combinations of herbs that contain not only iron but also the many other minerals that are vital for effective iron absorption. Liquid herbal iron tonics have long been available in health-food stores and are often recommended for new mothers. They are a convenient way to rebuild your blood.

Tonic or "adaptogenic" herbs are another possibility. (The term "adaptogenic" refers to herbs that can help you adapt to stresses that may be causing a variety of medical conditions.) These herbs alleviate fatigue, exhaustion, sleeplessness, and a general feeling of being run-down. They are often used preventively to keep illness at bay. In general, tonics are used daily for long periods of time. Adaptogenic herbs contain dozens of plant chemicals, each of which have unique and beneficial (but often weak) effects on their own. Their mode of action isn't fully understood.

In Asia and in Traditional Chinese Medicine, the many species of ginseng (Chinese, Korean, and American ginseng) are used in tonics. All are members of the genus *Panax*. Be aware that the term "ginseng" is often erroneously applied to any herb that has a tonic effect. For example, eleuthero is called Siberian ginseng but is not a true ginseng. Even the Ayurvedic tonic herb known as ashwagandha is sometimes called Indian ginseng. A true, or *Panax*, ginseng has an overall stimulating effect, though it isn't a stimulant like coffee. Ginsengs help you feel more energetic; however, they are also known to increase blood pressure.

Eleuthero, or Siberian ginseng, lacks the stimulating effects of true ginsengs. Eleuthero isn't known or expected to affect breastfeeding babies. Ashwagandha is considered a sedative tonic, meaning it is relaxing as well as energizing, and it helps to relieve fatigue and build stamina in daily life. In India, ashwagandha is considered to be a galactogogue, especially when combined with other herbs.

The true ginsengs and other tonic herbs such as wu wei zi (schisandra) and rhodiola have been extensively studied in Asia and Russia. The plants are thought to have a whole host of helpful effects on the body. There are no anecdotes, as yet, to suggest that they will affect breast-feeding babies. Ginseng is used in China with nursing women who suffer postpartum exhaustion or mastitis—but only after careful diagnosis within the paradigm of Traditional Chinese Medicine.

In Asia, postpartum women are commonly given Chinese angelica, or dong quai, typically in soups made with bones (an excellent source of calcium and other minerals). According to one report, a woman became dizzy and both she and her baby developed high blood pressure after the woman consumed soup that was believed to contain dong quai. The health of both soon returned to normal, however, and the soup was never analyzed to determine its contents. Because dong quai is known to lower blood pressure, this incident remains a mystery.

Other excellent and commonly used tonics are garlic and ginger. In Asia, large amounts of these herbs are eaten every day as part of a delicious diet. Other than allergy and sensitivity to garlic in mother or baby, there is little reason to avoid these strengthening herbs. Note that garlic and ginger may slow blood clotting. Avoid medicinal use if you are already on blood thinners.

Other tonics—such as the delicious Chinese medicinal mushrooms reishi and shiitake, for example—are commonly used and available in stores nationwide. Mushrooms, like seaweeds, need to be raised in environments free of heavy metal contamination. Astragalus, a member of the pea family, may be helpful as a tonic, too. Daily use of astragalus during cold and flu season can help prevent illness. Astragalus isn't associated with allergic reactions.

Wounds, Bruises, and Skin Problems

Wounds, burns, and bruises, as well as other skin problems like eczema and psoriasis, are often treated herbally with external applications.

When applied over unbroken skin, herbs and properly diluted essential oils aren't expected to cause problems during breastfeeding—as long as such applications aren't on or near the breasts. Keeping your baby's hands and mouth away from treatment areas will ensure that he won't ingest anything he shouldn't.

Special care is needed if you use topical capsicum or capsaicin products for nerve pain or arthritic conditions. Capsaicin is basically the hot stuff in cayenne peppers. Getting it into your eyes is very unpleasant. Even if capsaicin doesn't cause actual tissue damage, it can be extremely irritating. The last thing you want to do is expose your baby to it. You need to scrub hard with soap and water to remove the hot stuff from your hands. Test if it's been fully removed by putting your fingers in your mouth after scrubbing—any tingling? If so, then scrub again. Consider using disposable rubber gloves during each application.

There are many wound-healing herbs that are nontoxic and non-allergenic. Selection depends on what sort of skin problem you have, so consult a good herbal book first. Penelope Ody's book *The Complete Medicinal Herbal* (see appendix A) is a helpful guide.

Bruises heal more quickly when arnica oil or St. John's wort oil (both made by infusion) is applied to them. Note that homeopathic arnica can be used internally to heal bruises and wounds.

The external application of nontoxic herbs and essential oils on intact skin isn't expected to affect lactation or your baby. However, you may react with allergic dermatitis or other skin irritations. Essential oils especially need to be used in an appropriate manner: at the proper dilution in carrier oils. Never assume that you can use just any essential oil straight. Many oils are extremely irritating in concentration. Oregano, for example, may be a familiar herb, but oregano essential oil can make your skin peel if the oil hasn't been properly diluted. (Read more about essential oils in chapter 4.) Always be aware of an essential oil's potential for skin irritation, allergic reaction, and toxicity.

Open wounds require more caution, as absorption of plant constituents into the body is much greater through open wounds than intact skin. Using potentially toxic herbs such as arnica oil or crude comfrey root on open wounds isn't recommended by most herbalists and plant toxicology experts. Keep in mind that sore nipples are essentially open wounds, as are tears or incisions around the perineum. For more about the care of sore nipples, see chapter 8. In chapter 6, you'll find a discussion about proper care of stitches and tears around the perineum.

Avoid using toxic or irritating herbs on or near mucous membranes: the nipples, mouth, nose, anus, labia, and vagina. Mucous membranes are thinner than skin and therefore more able to absorb plant constituents. Why risk an allergic or irritated skin reaction in these tender areas? Seek safer alternatives and gentler remedies.

A final note: Skin rashes, infected wounds (red, hot and throbbing, oozing, painful), or any mysterious skin conditions that don't respond quickly to home treatments—whether herbal or over-the-counter—should be evaluated by a doctor.

Weight-Loss Issues

Our society tells us that, as women, we need to be slim and trim at all times, and we certainly shouldn't let a little thing like having a baby derail us from having the "perfect" feminine form. The pressure to quickly regain our pre-pregnant size and shape runs counter to our biology, however. Some weight gain during pregnancy is normal and healthy. After birth, you need calories as you produce milk for your child—so, it seems that Mother Nature adds those curves for a good reason.

To maintain a healthy caloric intake while you're nursing, all you've got to do is add the amount of calories in a peanut butter sandwich (no more, no less) to your daily diet, and you'll have the right amount of extra calories you need. Many mothers naturally add these calories to their diet because breastfeeding tends to increase their appetites. As the months go by, the pounds will start slipping away, despite the extra calories you consume, especially if you eat nutritious, satisfying foods in reasonable portions. Some women find that the most dramatic weight loss comes in the second year of breastfeeding and, unlike after dieting, this weight stays off. It's true that some women don't lose their pregnancy weight while breastfeeding—but most do. Trust in breastfeeding to help you lose that weight, but stick to eating wholesome foods in reasonable amounts. Breastfeeding isn't a miracle diet. No such thing exists.

Dieting in the first year of breastfeeding is unnecessary and counterproductive. From your baby's point of view, any body fat you've got is future breast milk just waiting to be enjoyed. Get comfortable with your curvy figure, and don't expect to return to your pre-pregnant shape right away. The weight loss will come as a natural consequence of breastfeeding. Although you may not initially lose weight while breastfeeding, studies have shown that after the first year, you can expect to weigh less than those who didn't breastfeed or who weaned early.

Crash dieting, or severely restricting your food intake, affects your level of nutrition and energy (although not necessarily your baby's). Besides drawing on your fat stores, your body is using many other nutrients to make milk—nutrients that are best replaced every day. If you don't feed your body well, it will let you know—and all the more quickly when breastfeeding. It's hard enough to get sufficient rest as a new mom, so why invite the double whammy of additional fatigue as a result of not feeding yourself?

Severe dieting forces the body to metabolize stored fats, which leads to the release of toxins from the stored fats. All mammals have toxins stored in fats (an unfortunate fact of modern life). These toxins are absorbed over a lifetime and mobilized during breastfeeding. Rapid weight loss will result in the faster release of such toxins, increasing the amount entering your milk. Keep in mind that the amounts of toxins released into the milk are extremely tiny. Still, this is another reason to avoid sudden weight loss from crash dieting.

Before you start to worry about toxins in your milk, know this: The fact that your baby is being exposed to these toxins doesn't mean you should quit breastfeeding. The risks of formula feeding far outweigh the potential risks of these toxins. If there's any doubt in your mind, take a look at chapter 1 for a review of the benefits of feeding your baby breast milk.

You've probably noticed that natural health magazines are often crammed with ads promising rapid weight loss. Some of the advertised products are simply ineffective, but others are potentially dangerous. In general, the use of such weight-loss products is not recommended, for a variety of reasons. Many contain certain herbs or herbal combinations that can negatively affect you, your baby, and even breastfeeding itself.

A number of well-known weight-loss products contain the herb ephedra, also called *ma huang*. This herb contains the plant chemicals ephedrine, pseudoephedrine, and other closely related compounds, collectively called ephedra alkaloids. These chemicals act as stimulants to the nervous system. (Weight loss is known to occur with most nervous stimulants, herbal or pharmaceutical.) While the stimulant herb ephedra and its constituent chemicals have bona fide traditional and conventional medicinal uses, they cannot be recommended for nursing mothers. A number of over-the-counter medications for colds and hay fever also contain pseudoephedrine, or even the more powerful ephedrine, so always check the ingredient lists. In sufficient doses, ephedrine can cause overstimulation in breastfed babies.

Many weight-loss products use a combination of stimulant herbs—ephedra and caffeine-containing herbs being the most common. Guarana, yerba maté, kola nut, coffee, and black tea all contain caffeine. Caffeine is known to overstimulate some breastfeeding babies, especially newborns. The combination of ephedra and caffeine would likely be too much for your breastfeeding baby—and possibly for you, too. This is why some experts consider ephedra products to be dangerous. Cases of serious adverse effects in adults have almost always involved combination products, and not caffeine or ephedra alone. (The most serious cases occurred when large doses were followed by physical exertion.) While such combination products aren't likely to provide a big enough dose to permanently harm an infant, they are likely to leave him unable to sleep or crying for hours on end. And the products are likely to have you dry-mouthed, jittery, and wound up yourself.

Ephedra also has the potential to affect your milk supply. In a recent carefully conducted human study, pseudoephedrine was shown to lower milk supply. This finding supports what many mothers have noticed for years—that their milk supply drops when they use products containing pseudoephedrine. Mothers need to be especially cautious about ephedra alkaloids in the early weeks of lactation, a time when milk supply is being established. You should avoid over-the-counter extended release forms (twelve and twenty-four hour) of pseudoephedrine in particular. Even though it isn't as powerful as ephedrine, the effects of pseudoephedrine can extend over several nursing sessions.

Manufacturers of herbal weight-loss products are moving away from using ephedra, but often this means they've substituted other stimulating herbs. For example, country mallow, or flannelweed *(Sida cordifolia)*, and bitter orange don't have ephedrine, but do contain other naturally occurring stimulants. Some unscrupulous manufacturers now use such plants while advertising their products as "ephedra-free"—so, buyer beware. Many such products also contain hefty doses of caffeine and caffeine-containing herbs.

Elimination Problems (Bladder, Bowel)

Bladder infections are common during pregnancy and are thought to be related to high levels of certain hormones. Bladder infections can also occur soon after birth, especially if you had to be catheterized during or after delivery. Cranberry juice is the first line of defense. Drinking at least 8 oz. of sweetened, mixed cranberry juice a day, or 6 oz. of pure cranberry juice a day, has been shown to help clear an infection. There is no need to wait for an infection, however; cranberry juice can be used preventively as well.

Eating yogurt or taking probiotics (encapsulated acidophilus and other "good guy" bacteria) can help re-establish or maintain a good mix of intestinal flora. This seems to help prevent bladder infections, too. Dehydration can contribute to these infections. Don't let yourself get dehydrated, something that can easily happen after nursing a lot at night. Keeping water by the bedside helps.

Mothers often experience constipation after birth. It may be only a temporary situation, not requiring any medicinal herbs other than plenty of fresh fruits and vegetables, stewed prunes, bran, or perhaps psyllium (found in products such as Metamucil). If you tend to become constipated, drink some fluids every time you nurse, including at night.

If you become dehydrated, your stool may become harder. An herbalist may be able to suggest mild laxative herbs that are also considered beneficial in the postpartum. For example, both yellow dock and dandelion root have a mild laxative effect and are also used to "build up the blood" after hemorrhage in childbirth. They are not known to cause cramps or diarrhea. Make sure the basics of bowel management are covered: a healthy diet with lots of roughage, plenty of fluids, and a good amount of exercise. In particular, yoga can do wonders for bowel regulation.

Herbalists have long known that giving a mother stimulant laxative herbs can have distressing effects on the young infant, and a typical herb book will advise against any use of these herbs for nursing mothers. On the other hand, the American Academy of Pediatrics has approved the use of the over-the-counter herbs cascara and senna and their derivatives during lactation. Why the difference? It's mostly a matter of dose. Over-the-counter herbal laxatives deliver a predictable dose of their herbal constituents. At commonly recommended dosages, none of these active constituents make it into the breast milk. Keep in mind that, in higher doses, the laxative constituents can spill into the breast milk and may cause diarrhea in very young infants. According to Varro Tyler's book *Herbs of Choice,* cascara is the gentlest of the stimulant laxative herbs. Senna leaf and fruit are cheaper, and, as a result, OTC senna products are more easily found in stores.

Stick to OTC cascara and senna products that specify the dose of active ingredients right on the label, and don't exceed the listed dose. If you really don't want to use over-the-counter pills, it's possible to purchase tea bags with standardized amounts of cascara bark and senna leaf. Some brands are made to over-the-counter specifications. These products often use cascara or senna in combination with herbs known to make the product gentler (and better tasting, too). To prepare a proper dose, carefully follow the instructions for how much water to use and how long to steep the tea.

If your child is especially sensitive to senna, try a fraction of the suggested dose at first and watch your baby for any signs of cramps or loose stool. Use only as much as needed, in the smallest dose that is effective, and over as short a time as possible. Do not use a stimulant laxative for more than one to two weeks, as this can make your bowels dependent on them. Stimulant laxatives also cause a loss of potassium. If you take licorice or certain drugs along with laxatives, it is possible to develop a potassium deficiency. Stimulant laxatives shouldn't be used when abdominal pain or swelling is present, or if you have Crohn's disease, colitis, or other gastrointestinal conditions where inflammation may be present.

Some stimulant laxative herbs are much more likely to cause cramping and diarrhea than others and should be avoided. Alder buckthorn, purging buckthorn, rhubarb root, Chinese rhubarb, and aloes (but not aloe gel) are all considered stronger than cascara sagrada and senna; these can easily provoke cramping. The most powerful laxative herbs are called purgatives and once were extensively used in conventional medicine as "cure-alls" (if they didn't kill you first). Thankfully, those days are gone, and the use of herbs such as jalap, purging croton, and the infamous scammony is historic. (For the most part, that is; I have occasionally seen these herbs offered for sale.) Laxative herbs are not all the same. See appendix C for the safety ratings of the herbs mentioned in this section. Consult an herbalist before using any bulk product or a combination product that contains stimulant laxatives.

Thyroid Problems

If you are chronically fatigued, have a poor appetite, feel depressed, or are struggling with low milk supply, you need to see a physician to have your thyroid function checked. These symptoms are all associated with low thyroid function.

Low thyroid is treated with hormone replacement, either from natural sources (desiccated thyroid) or synthetic thyroid medication (Synthroid, for example). The supplements simply bring your thyroid hormones to a normal level. Both treatments are considered by the American Academy of Pediatrics to be compatible with breastfeeding, so there is no reason to wean even a small infant during use. Note that, according to lactation expert Dr. Ruth Lawrence, if you're diagnosed as hypothyroid (abnormally low thyroid function), your baby should also be checked for low thyroid.

You may have been told that your thyroid is working in the normal range but near low levels (borderline). With borderline thyroid function, doctors are reluctant to prescribe thyroid replacement, as there isn't clear evidence of medical need. Borderline low thyroid, despite looking normal to a physician, often doesn't feel normal to a woman who may feel tired all the time, even with adequate sleep. There are alternative treatments for improving the function of the sluggish or low-normal thyroid.

Many herbalists suggest seaweeds, as they are rich sources of iodine and other nutritional minerals. Though low iodine levels are unlikely to develop because of our modern iodized salt-rich diets, some people do suffer from this problem. Strict avoidance of salt (especially when coupled with diets rich in foods such as soybeans, beans, and certain other vegetables known to slow thyroid function) may result in iodine insufficiency. Soy formula for babies, for example, must be fortified with iodine to prevent thyroid suppression. Of course, seaweeds contain more than minerals; they are rich in complex cellulose-like materials unique to the plant world. These mucilaginous compounds aren't digested and so remain in the GI tract where they may slow down iodine absorption. It isn't known at this time how much of the iodine in seaweeds is actually absorbed into the body or how much seaweed you would need to eat to increase the iodine levels in breast milk. But some experts have cautioned breastfeeding women against using them. This caution may be well intentioned, as iodine does concentrate in breast milk; too much will suppress thyroid function in the baby. However, this doesn't seem to occur even in places like Japan, where seaweeds are eaten daily by nursing mothers. There is a great need for more research on the relationship between thyroid function, seaweeds, and iodine. At this time, there is much speculation and few facts to guide recommendations.

If you do use seaweeds, be sure that they have been collected from unpolluted waters. All seaweeds—but especially the brown seaweeds like kelp and bladder wrack—are able to concentrate heavy metals such as cadmium, mercury, and lead from seawater.

Ironically, overwhelming fatigue can also be a symptom of an overactive thyroid as well as low thyroid function. Other symptoms of an overactive thyroid may include irritability, nervous tension, heart palpitations, rapid weight loss, and insomnia. It is fairly common for women to develop an overactive thyroid three to six months postpartum (postpartum thyroiditis). The condition doesn't require medical treatment, as it typically goes away by itself in six to ten weeks. However, this condition must be distinguished from the true hyperthyroid condition known as Graves' disease, which is serious and absolutely requires medical treatment. Symptoms of an overactive thyroid should always be investigated by a doctor. A simple blood test will determine if the thyroid is overactive.

In many cases, physicians will want to rule out Graves' disease using a special radioactive iodine scan. For nursing mothers, such a scan isn't recommended, as the radioactive iodine will enter breast milk and is likely to cause harm to the baby. Mothers would have to stop breastfeeding, then pump and dump their milk for several days—a situation that has often led to weaning, breast infections, and emotional trauma to both mother and baby. Physicians with expertise in lactation tend to view this test as unnecessary, as most postpartum women with overactive thyroid will return to normal after a few weeks without treatment. Some physicians suggest alternative treatment with propranolol to improve symptoms. If symptoms don't improve after several weeks and blood tests continue to show signs of Graves' disease, doctors will initiate the standard drug treatment: propylthiouracil (PTU). This treatment is considered compatible with breastfeeding by the American Academy of Pediatrics.

Several herbs have long been used to affect thyroid function, most notably bugleweed (*Lycopus* species). While some herbalists believe that bugleweed can normalize thyroid function—speed it up when it's sluggish or slow it down when it's overactive—scientists consider the herb to be specifically antithyroid. Experiments have also shown the herb to have an antiprolactin effect, so nursing mothers are encouraged to avoid bugleweed. Herbal experts are reluctant to suggest antithyroid herbs for treating thyroid conditions in breastfeeding women.

If you have been diagnosed with overactive thyroid, you need a doctor to oversee your care until the problem is resolved. Thyroid problems definitely need careful medical attention. To safely treat a thyroid condition with herbs, it is necessary to find a medical herbalist and a physician who are willing to coordinate care. Nursing mothers need expert care, given the complexity of the thyroid and its role in maintaining milk supply. At present, there is very little research to guide herbal thyroid therapies for nursing mothers.

Postpartum Depression

In traditional cultures, postpartum depression is rare. These societies honor the new mother and attend to her for an extended period of time after birth. Special foods, healing rituals, and a suspension of her usual responsibilities all underscore the mother's newly elevated status and demonstrate her importance to the group. The mother gets plenty of rest, good food, and expert teaching on how to look after herself and the new baby. It's possible that the special foods and herbs given in traditional societies help new mothers get through postpartum hormonal changes with less angst.

In modern societies, mothers who don't have this support and who aren't honored by those around them often suffer depression and anxiety. We do know that a startling number of new mothers in modern society seek relief for depression, anxiety, and insomnia in the first year or so of their baby's life.

To treat postpartum depression, many doctors fall back on an all-too-standard approach—antidepressants—and advise mothers to wean in order to start treatment. (Ironically, mothers often feel that breastfeeding is the one thing in their lives that is going well.) Lactation experts generally believe that not only is weaning a poor solution to the problem of depression, it might make matters even worse. Some pediatricians are reluctant to prescribe antidepressants to nursing mothers, as these drugs may potentially affect the baby's developing brain, although this effect has yet to be demonstrated. What is known for sure is that untreated depression in the mother does affect the mental and emotional

St. John's Wort *(Hypericum perforatum)*

A number of herbs have been used to alleviate depression, St. John's wort (SJW) being the most studied and widely used. This herb blooms around the twenty-fourth of June, St. John's Day—hence, its name. Its bright yellow blossoms are commonly seen over much of North America, though it is considered an undesirable weed in agriculture.

The flowering tops of this plant have long been used to treat mild to moderate depressive states (but not severe depression). SJW has few side effects. To date, there are no published records of any adverse reactions in breastfeeding infants. One mother has reported that within a few days of starting a typical dose of SJW for depression, her four-month-old baby became fussy at the breast and began to choke and cry. When the mother stopped taking SJW, her baby's symptoms quickly went away. It's possible that SJW was making her let-down reflex stronger and her baby was reacting to the heavier flow of milk. St. John's wort oil has been used on the breasts to stimulate let-down when engorgement is present; however, recent studies have shown that SJW actually lowers prolactin temporarily (in rats, mind you); but after a few weeks—about the time it starts to take effect—prolactin levels rise to higher levels than before treatment. There are no lactation studies as yet.

St. John's wort has an advantage over pharmaceuticals in that it produces fewer side effects; this means it is less likely to produce effects in baby, too. Unlike pharmaceuticals, though, different brands of SJW can vary in quality and effectiveness. Look for standardized products made in Germany; these have formal studies backing their safety and efficacy. Note that some women find that the typical suggested dose is too high, resulting in their becoming "hyper." Use the smallest dose that works. If you're interested in SJW, be sure to talk to an herbal expert for more information about dosage levels and duration of use. If one of your symptoms development of her child. Yet a treatment that requires weaning may be equally harmful, since the nutrition that formula provides for a growing baby's brain and body is much inferior to that of mother's milk.

In short, depression must be treated. But what is the best treatment? Antidepressant medications can help with severe depression, and several are considered compatible with breastfeeding. Prozac is a less desirable option, as it has been found to have some side effects on breastfeeding babies. But other antidepressants have had few effects on breastfed infants.

The safest treatment is cognitive therapy (a specific form of counseling), which is known to quickly and effectively improve the symptoms of even severe postpartum depression. If you choose this option, find out if you can bring your baby with you during counseling sessions so you can continue bonding and breastfeeding as you talk through the issues that are affecting you. Getting emotional support from other people in your life can help, too. When you have attentive family members and friends around you, you're more likely to feel nourished and supported.

Changing your diet may help improve your mood. Studies have shown, for example, that eating a nonprotein snack before bedtime increases serotonin levels in the brain. La Leche League's web site has many excellent articles by the psychologist Kathleen Kendall-Tackett describing how dietary, herbal, and cognitive therapies can be useful in treating postpartum depression. A La Leche League Leader can also provide you with these and other articles.

Herbal allies can play an important part in overcoming postpartum depression. Melissa, or lemon balm, is known as "the gladdening herb." A couple of cups of fragrant lemon balm tea can lift the spirits, and so can a number of other teas: chamomile, lavender, and rose. Blessed thistle tea (one or two cups per day) can help relieve postpartum depression, though in larger amounts it may increase your milk supply. The most famous and by far the most extensively studied of these herbal allies is St. John's wort (see the previous page).

If you're depressed, seeking out other mothers allows you to share your feelings and hear what other women in a similar situation have experienced. La Leche League Leaders or other lactation specialists can help you connect with nursing mothers who have gone through post-partum depression and can recommend local support groups that will support your breastfeeding efforts.

Insomnia and Lack of Sleep

Everyone is different when it comes to sleep. Some people are convinced that they can't live without eight hours or more of sleep a night; others know from experience that they can survive on short snatches of sleep for several days in a row, as long as they get at least three or four hours of rest in there somewhere. The main difference between these groups is that the people in the first one haven't had children yet.

As you know, life with a baby often means a life without a lot of sleep. It can be helpful to nap when your baby naps; this can help balance out all those sleep interruptions at night. But if you work during the day or are taking care of other children, naps may be few and far between.

If you find yourself wakeful during the night, you may wonder if taking a sleep aid would be safe. Talk to your doctor about a prescription sleep aid or even the short-term use of an over-the-counter medication; these drugs can be quite powerful and may not be safe to take if you are "co-sleeping" with your baby. If you prefer herbal sleep remedies, nervines (herbs that help you relax) such as oats, chamomile, valerian, passionflower, hops, lemon balm, kava, and skullcap are possibilities. While individual sensitivity to these nervines varies, most people who use nervines don't feel "dopey" if woken up during the night, nor do they feel hung over in the morning.

Not all nervines are equally safe, however. Here is some important information on those that are most commonly used:

- Oats (oat straw), chamomile, and occasional use of passionflower are generally without controversy. Oat straw, either as a tea or as a glycerite preparation, is reputed to build up the nervous system and help with general nervousness or stress-related symptoms.

- When using chamomile for sleep, use two tea bags per 6 oz. of water; the tea should be allowed to steep for only 2–3 minutes in a tightly covered container. For those allergic to ragweed, there is some risk of allergic reactions with Roman chamomile; German chamomile is much less allergenic.

- Hops are considered galactogogues when used in teas or tinctures, meaning they may increase milk supply. (See chapter 7 for milk supply issues.) Hops are often used in sleep pillows; the strobiles (flower structures) will give off a relaxing scent for about a week.

- Lemon balm *(Melissa officinalis)*, "the gladdening herb," is also called "the scholar's herb," as it helps improve memory and thinking. Like chamomile, the tea at bedtime aids sleep. Lemon balm has also been used as a mild galactogogue.

- Valerian is widely used as a sleep aid. It has been shown to shorten the time it takes to get to sleep, to help sleep return if awakened, and to lengthen sleep time. It smells really bad (some people think it smells like stinky socks), so you probably won't want to try the tea. Consider valerian capsules instead. Although valerian is known to contain potentially toxic compounds called valepotriates, these chemicals are poorly absorbed and rapidly break down to less toxic compounds almost immediately after valerian is picked. There are no reports of adverse reactions in babies. The plant is often used with children, especially in England, and does not cause toxicity. Continual use of valerian can cause headaches and, ironically, insomnia and agitation in some people, however.

- Kava *(Piper methysticum)* has been shown to relax the muscles, which can be helpful when trying to get to sleep. Kava use during breastfeeding is controversial, however, as discussed in the following section on anxiety.

- Skullcap (*Scutellaria* species) is often cited in herbal books for relieving anxiety and inducing sleep. There is a big problem with this herb though, as a lot of products labeled "skullcap" are adulterated with another herb called germander *(Teucrium chamaedrys)*, which is known to be toxic. There are numerous reports of skullcap products causing liver damage, and even experts cannot determine if all are due to germander or not. For safety, it is best to avoid skullcap products.

Anxiety

If you're suffering from anxiety, it may be that you're overwhelmed with the typical worries and concerns that come with motherhood. On the other hand, anxiety is, for some people, a more serious problem. Talk to your healthcare provider about your symptoms; it may also be helpful to reach out to your breastfeeding supporters (see chapter 2).

You may have heard about the herb kava, which has been used as a relaxant. Traditional societies throughout the South Pacific and Hawaii use kava medicinally and in social rituals. In Hawaiian tradition, adults, children, and infants are treated with kava for various health problems. Kava has more recently been used in Western cultures for the treatment of anxiety, sleeplessness, and muscle spasms. Controlled studies of kava have found it to be an effective treatment for anxiety. Therapeutic doses are neither sedating nor addictive. But kava in very high doses (overdose) is capable of sedating an adult.

With regard to breastfeeding, kava is the most widely contraindicated herb in both medical and herbalist literature. There are no known adverse events involving breastfed babies, even though some nursing mothers use kava. However, recent cases of liver damage associated with German kava products have provoked the German government to take kava off the market. No similar cases have been found in the United States.

A possible explanation for this toxicity is that certain kava producers may be using the stems as well as the rhizomes to provide adequate supplies to certain German herbal manufacturers. The stems have recently been found to contain liver toxins. Some popular German kava products are also twice as concentrated as those in the United States. So far, kava rhizome products in the United States are not known to have produced toxic effects. Even so, kava products must be viewed with some caution, as they may vary in quality. Those with liver impairment or who use other medications should talk with a knowledgeable physician before using kava. If treatment of anxiety is medically necessary, it is best to discuss the benefits and hazards of kava versus tranquilizing pharmaceuticals such as benzodiazepines. Tranquilizers have disadvantages: they are sedating, they are addictive, and they have been known to sedate infants (as, for example, in the case of Valium). Kava has none of these disadvantages, though it shouldn't be taken with alcohol. Kava safety is a hot topic at present, so consider your treatment choices carefully. Seek the help of your breastfeeding and herbal experts before self-treating with kava.

Migraines

For some women, breastfeeding seems to prevent migraines. Others see no difference in the level of their migraines, and some women find that their migraines are worse or more frequent. Rarely, some nursing mothers experience a brief migraine upon let-down of their milk. For those who suffer migraines, medical options are somewhat limited.

There are a number of drugs that are used for migraine headaches, some of which can be used when breastfeeding. The oldest drugs, called ergot alkaloids (for example, ergotamine) are contraindicated during the first months of breastfeeding because they suppress prolactin, which, as a result, greatly lowers milk supply. These drugs can occasionally be used later in breastfeeding (when the baby is older), however. Beta-blockers and tricyclic antidepressants have been used, though they have side effects that can affect nursing mothers. Sumatriptan is a drug specifically used to treat a migraine attack; it has some serious, if rare, side effects that many find unacceptable. None of the medications commonly used for migraine are known to affect breastfeeding babies, as the amount of the drugs entering the breast milk is very small. The level of treatment you need will greatly depend on the frequency and severity of your headaches.

One herb has been found to help prevent migraines when taken daily: feverfew. The preferable dose is one fresh leaf chewed and swallowed. Feverfew grows easily in gardens, and in warmer climates it's possible to have a nearly year-round supply of fresh leaves. Unfortunately, the active constituents of feverfew (parthenolides) are easily broken down after picking, so that many feverfew products have been found to contain no active constituents at all. This makes choosing a good quality product that much more important; if one doesn't work, try another, as it may just have been a bad product. Look for a product that is standardized to contain a guaranteed amount of parthenolides.

Feverfew has no known or expected adverse effects on lactation or on breastfeeding babies. The plant is in the daisy family, however, so some people will be allergic to it. Mouth sores sometimes develop with use and can occur even when the leaf is swallowed in capsule form. These sores apparently go away after a few weeks of continued treatment. Feverfew will not help a migraine already in progress. But because feverfew can prevent an attack, you probably won't have to use the more powerful drugs as often.

One natural remedy for stopping a migraine is to inhale a few grains of cayenne pepper through the nose. (Note: Do this carefully with only a few grains, an amount small enough to be picked up on a toothpick.) I am told this hurts in the nose like crazy for a short time but can stop a migraine, especially if caught early enough. A strong cup of espresso may also help in the midst of an attack.

Rubbing the temples with lavender oil or other essential oils can help relieve migraine pain. This is something you can do while you wait for the stronger analgesics to kick in. Learn about these essential oils and any sensitivities you may have before using them. While most herbs that are used externally are not considered to be risky during breastfeeding, it is wise to know which essential oils may be allergenic or irritating if used at full strength.

Varicose Veins and Hemorrhoids

Varicose veins typically start during pregnancy and can persist in the postpartum. Some women don't get them, while others are severely affected. Varicose veins tend to run in families.

The cause? The walls of the veins in the legs, as well as in the rectum and anus, become thin and relax; the vessels then swell. At first, you may see a spider web of tiny veins appearing on the legs, and eventually the large vessels may start to stick out and get bumpy with knots. These are signs that blood is pooling in the veins and it is getting harder and harder for the body to move the blood up out of the legs against gravity. This back pressure of blood causes fluid to leak out of the tiniest blood vessels in the legs, the capillaries, and into the surrounding tissues. The ankles and lower legs puff up, and painful aching ensues. Varicose veins in the rectum are called hemorrhoids. Hemorrhoids will swell, ache, and may even break and bleed when you are passing stool.

Wearing loose clothing that doesn't bind the legs and wearing supportive stockings (for example, TED hose or compression stockings) are the mainstays of treatment, regardless of what other therapies are used. Avoid socks with elastic tops, tight pants, and tight panties. Staying off your feet can help, a luxury for most mothers. Nursing is a good excuse to sit down, so put your feet up and enjoy the rest. Better yet, lie down with your legs up as high as you can get them (perhaps on a wall or chair). Once you relieve the pressure, fluid can circulate out of the legs; the swelling goes down, and the ache goes away.

Cold compresses can relieve swelling veins. You can make cold compresses using calendula flowers, hawthorn berries, wild violet leaves, or witch hazel bark and leaf. Make a strong tea and chill it before use. Soak cold cloths in the tea, then apply them to the swelling veins. You can also apply commercial witch hazel, which comes in a bottle. Witch hazel is widely used for hemorrhoids and is often an ingredient in commercial hemorrhoid relief pads. Consider applying cold compresses as you sit down to nurse. It helps to sit or lie down with your feet up every couple of hours, whether you're nursing at the time or not.

Breastfeeding and Diabetes

Sometimes, mothers are discouraged from breastfeeding because they have diabetes. However, insulin-dependent diabetic mothers have found that the disease is generally easier to control while they are nursing and they require less insulin. Further, babies exclusively breastfed in the early months have a lower risk of developing diabetes.

If you are diabetic, you may be interested in exploring herbs that complement drug treatments for high blood sugar. Be aware that herbs that lower blood sugar or increase insulin sensitivity should be used under careful medical supervision. Among the better-studied anti-diabetic herbs are gymnema and fenugreek. Combining these herbs with oral antidiabetic medications can be problematic; these drugs are considered less desirable for use during breastfeeding anyway. A number of widely used galactogogue (milk-increasing) herbs may lower blood sugar in modest amounts, an effect that may actually be advantageous to diabetic mothers with low milk supply.

Circulation-stimulating herbs such as ginger, as well as water-releasing dandelion leaves, are often suggested to help move fluid out of the legs. You can drink them as a tea or include them in your diet.

One of the best-known and researched herbal remedies for varicose veins is horse chestnut. A well-manufactured product would be standardized to contain 16 to 20 percent aescin, the constituent that is most responsible for making the veins less "leaky." In Germany, a delayed-release capsule called Venastat has been shown effective and safe for treating varicose veins. Any side effects, drug interactions, or contraindications for its use have yet to be identified. There are also no expected or known adverse effects with breastfeeding, according to the German Commission E. Venastat is stocked in many pharmacies.

Do not use crude, unprocessed forms of horse chestnut, as these are toxic. (Children have been poisoned by eating raw horse chestnuts.) The controlled dose of the delayed-release capsule ensures safety. There is also a horse chestnut cream that can be applied to the legs. It is not readily available in the United States, however.

Foods rich in vitamin C, the flavonoid rutin, lecithin, and vitamin E are particularly helpful for varicose veins. For more vitamin C, eat whole oranges instead of drinking orange juice. The white part of citrus rinds is especially rich in rutin, as are wild violets, which are up to 23 percent rutin. If you have these flowers in your yard, you can make a tea or compress (or simply apply the fresh leaves as a compress). Dried wild violet leaves and flowers can be made into tea as well. Just don't consume large quantities of the leaves, as they may make you nauseated. Garlic, onions, chives, and leeks are rich sources of quercetin, another flavonoid that strengthens capillaries. The peel of the onion or garlic is the best source of quercetin—and is perfect for making soup stock.

Bilberry and other dark red berries rich in anthocyanidin pigments help vitamin C do its job. The dark red and blue pigments in these berries are known to reduce the fragility of the capillaries and can help prevent swelling. So feast on blueberries, cranberries, cherries, and bilberries—the darker the better. Of course, if you eat too many, you may get diarrhea.

If you're not allergic to peanuts, the papery skins of Spanish peanuts will also reduce capillary fragility and "leakiness." Peanuts are a much cheaper source than the commercial product known as Pycnogenol, and they contain the same important constituents—oligomeric procyanidins, or OPCs. Buckwheat, too, is remarkable for its ability to strengthen blood vessels. (Note: Buckwheat can cause severe allergenic reactions in some.)

Chronic Illness

It isn't uncommon for nursing mothers to be told that their health condition has been caused or worsened by breastfeeding. Mothers with certain chronic diseases may indeed suffer an exacerbation of the disease while breastfeeding. But can it be said for certain that breastfeeding was the cause?

Studies have determined that breastfeeding helps protect most, but not all, mothers from relapses of rheumatoid arthritis and multiple sclerosis. Further, studies have found that breastfeeding lowers the risk of baby's developing rheumatoid disease later in adulthood. Migraine sufferers cover the whole spectrum—from being well as long as they breastfeed to finding that let-downs can trigger an attack. Individual variability is the rule.

Sometimes, mothers are diagnosed with what appears to be a problem requiring drug treatment. For example, many mothers have been told they have high cholesterol and require medication, even though it is well known that blood cholesterol is normally elevated during lactation. Further, the medications typically used to treat high cholesterol aren't recommended while breastfeeding, as these drugs may interfere with the normal cholesterol formation needed for milk. If cholesterol medication is required, treatment does not need to begin immediately.

Chronic illness presents special challenges as there are no quick fixes or final cures. Some people search for anything that will make them feel better, and their desperation makes them vulnerable to overenthusiastic sales pitches for prescription drugs, miracle diets, and cure-all herbal products. Yet, more and more people are finding that simple dietary changes and certain dietary supplements do indeed make them feel better or reduce the need for prescription drugs. Of course, exercise can work wonders, and yoga and other disciplines that teach breath work are among the best forms of exercise for those with a chronic illness.

There are organizations, magazines, web sites, and support groups for just about any chronic condition. While you can educate yourself about the best alternative and complementary treatments for an illness, it is important to ask your doctor and other healthcare providers what they think about any self-administered remedies or treatment programs. If any source of information promises a cure or suggests that you stop following your doctor's advice—especially if it suggests that you stop taking a prescribed medication—view this information with suspicion. These are red flags and probably indicate an unreliable source.

When you ask your doctor his or her opinion about an alternative or complementary therapy, the response you receive should be serious and thoughtful, not off the top of the head or dismissive. For example, if you ask about specific dietary supplements, including herbs, an involved healthcare professional should research any potential safety issues related to the use of those supplements, as well as determine what evidence there is, if any, to support their use. He or she should tell you if your illness or condition precludes using any of these supplements and how the supplements might interact, if at all, with any prescribed medications you may be taking. Many herbs influence the actions of prescription drugs; some may increase the actions, while others may block them. You can sometimes work around these interactions by either increasing or decreasing the medication dose, but you will need your doctor's help to make these adjustments. In addition, herbs that increase the activity of a drug can sometimes be used to decrease the effective dose of that drug and, in the process, the risk of side effects from that drug.

This is new territory for most doctors, who will need the best information available to help you find consistently formulated herbal products with predictable effects. Contact the American Botanical Council (see appendix B) for the most up-to-date technical resources for your doctor and pharmacist.

A physician's oversight is especially important if you have impaired liver or kidney function, as certain foods and herbs can be irritating (or even toxic) to the liver or kidneys. In such cases, both the dose and duration of use of a remedy need to be monitored. Because prescription drugs can interact with foods and herbs, your doctor may have very good reasons for discouraging you from using a particular remedy while you are taking certain medications. While you may not agree with your doctor's assessment and may even have specific information to back up your position, it is important to share this information with the doctor and listen to his or her perspective. However, you do not have to tolerate a doctor's blanket dismissal of alternative and complementary therapies. Changing doctors or getting a second opinion is always your option as a patient.

As a nursing mother, you must carefully investigate new therapies before trying them. Many nursing mothers have asked me for help after seeing dubious treatments suggested on web sites, and sometimes I have uncovered good reasons for them to avoid such remedies—not necessarily because they would place their babies at risk, but because the herb under consideration wasn't the best choice for them. One mother of a two-year-old had poor kidney function and was asking about herbs that were known kidney irritants. The herbs posed a risk to the mother, not the toddler.

Numerous publications offer advice on alternative and complementary therapies for chronic illnesses. These books can be good starting points for investigation, but be sure to take with a grain of salt whatever they say about treatments during breastfeeding. Too often the concern is limited to the baby, who in most cases is not likely to be endangered by such therapies. A more likely risk is to breastfeeding itself, as many herbs can increase or decrease milk supply. Sometimes an herbal therapy can interact with prescription drugs that the mother needs to take or can worsen an existing medical condition. In most cases, safe alternative herbal therapies can be found with the help of an expert herbalist.

Chronic illnesses require expert assessment and the judicious use of treatments—pharmaceutical or herbal—whether you're breastfeeding or not. You need a team of professionals that can provide more guidance than what you'll find on the Internet or in health-food stores.

$\mathscr{W}$hen Your Baby Is Sick

At some point, your baby may become ill. This chapter offers some basic information on taking care of your sick baby. Note: This information is not intended as a substitute for professional medical attention. If your baby is sick, talk to your child's healthcare provider or bring him in for an evaluation.

Signs That Your Child Is Ill

When your baby isn't feeling well, he will most likely seek the comfort of your breast. In fact, your baby may want to nurse even if he is throwing up. If so, let him nurse. He may throw up again, but some of the milk will be digested. If he continues to throw up after nursing, consider offering him the breast he last nursed from; he will then get a smaller volume of milk, which is more likely to stay down. It's important to let your baby continue to nurse, so that he is less likely to become dehydrated.

If your baby is sick and refuses to nurse, you must take action immediately. Your child may be very sick indeed. Talk to your baby's doctor right away to find out if an office visit is needed. Sometimes, it's hard to know when to call the doctor. Any time that your baby doesn't seem quite "right" is a good time to call. Trust your instincts on this.

More specifically, always call the doctor if your baby:

- is lethargic or hard to rouse

- has a high fever

- cries inconsolably

- has a high-pitched cry

- isn't producing any wet diapers

All of these are signs of potentially serious illness. Don't delay in getting medical help.

Common Health Conditions

Spitting up (reflux), colic, constipation, blood in the stool, and sleep problems are common health conditions for many babies, whether or not they are breastfed. Know, however, that many doctors still suggest switching to baby formula to "solve" these health conditions, even though this is rarely necessary. Baby formula most likely won't help. In fact, it may worsen the problem.

Spitting Up

Spitting up may be normal, but projectile vomiting (throwing up forcefully) isn't. Call the doctor if your baby vomits forcefully. A serious medical problem may be the cause.

Some breastfed babies spit up a bit after every feeding yet are happy and continue to gain weight. Often, spitting up is more of a laundry problem than a medical problem and goes away as the baby matures. However, a very young baby who frequently spits up should be checked by a doctor.

Frequent spitting up may be a sign of reflux, but if the baby doesn't present any other symptoms, he probably doesn't have reflux. Babies with true reflux cannot keep their stomach acid from flowing back into the esophagus, which then becomes irritated and inflamed, causing pain. In severe cases, the stomach fluids may even flow into the lungs, causing breathing difficulties. Many babies with reflux don't spit anything up; the fluids just silently flow upward, causing problems.

Reflux is diagnosed with special tests, and treatment is aimed at keeping stomach acids in the stomach. If your baby has been diagnosed with reflux (or GERD), talk with a lactation specialist or other breastfeeding expert. There are good treatments for reflux that won't interfere with breastfeeding.

Switching to baby formula is often suggested in cases of reflux. However, reflux is usually worsened with formula feeding. If you continue to nurse your baby, it is wise to get help from a lactation expert who understands your situation.

You may have heard that thickening your breast milk with cereal and feeding this to your baby can help with reflux. Actually, studies have shown that this won't help and may even put your child at risk for an allergic reaction to the cereal. If your baby is very young, his digestive tract isn't mature enough to handle the added cereal.

In some cases, nursing mothers have found that making changes to their diet seemed to help their baby's reflux. Talk to a lactation specialist before trying this approach.

Colic

If your baby cries a lot or seems especially distressed after breastfeeding, you may wonder if he has colic. The good news is that he probably doesn't. Symptoms of colic are easily recognizable: unrelieved crying that can go on for hours and a constant pulling up of the legs—both reactions to abdominal pain. These signs leave no doubt that colic is the cause.

It isn't known exactly why colic occurs or why it often seems to magically disappear when a baby reaches about four months of age. Presumably, the baby's gut simply becomes more mature.

You may be told to wean if your baby has colic, but this isn't your only option. With a little detective work, you may be able to determine if your child is reacting to something in your diet (for example, cow's milk protein or orange juice). Or it may be that your baby is getting too much lactose and not enough of the fatty hind milk when he nurses. To solve this problem, let your baby empty one breast before you switch sides. In any case, contact a lactation specialist for tips on breastfeeding a colicky baby and getting through those difficult early months.

Many mothers of colicky babies look to herbal remedies for help. There are safe, effective ways to treat colic using herbs, but it's important to know what you're doing. Feeding herbs to an infant isn't always a good idea; there are safer ways to use herbs. See "Using Herbs Safely and Effectively" later in this chapter for a discussion of herbal treatments for colic.

Constipation

Constipation is rare when a baby is thriving on nothing but breast milk. However, at about six weeks of age, an exclusively breastfed baby may start to go many days (or even a couple of weeks) without moving his bowels. If your baby eventually produces a stool that is soft, then he is most likely fine and there is no cause for concern. But if constipation is accompanied by pain and cramping, there may be a problem. Call your doctor to talk about these symptoms.

When you begin to introduce solid foods to your baby (usually at around six months of age), his stool will become firmer and will have a more unpleasant smell. This is normal. If the stool becomes uncomfortably firm for your baby, work on increasing his intake of breast milk, which will help make the stool softer again. Your baby may find some foods to be more constipating than others. Keep a record of which foods have a more constipating effect, then reduce your baby's intake of them.

Bloody Stool

Blood in the stool is most often caused by a reaction to cow's milk protein. When the mother consumes foods containing cow's milk protein, small amounts of the protein can enter her breast milk. Babies who have blood in the stool after exposure to such small quantities of the protein are typically extremely sensitive to it. It may be risky to expose these babies to foods containing the protein.

If your baby is highly sensitive to cow's milk protein, delay introducing dairy products into his diet until he reaches about eighteen months of age. Meanwhile, eliminate cow's milk protein from your own diet for at least a couple of weeks. Talk to a lactation expert for guidance. Despite what you may have been told by a doctor, it usually isn't necessary or beneficial to switch your baby to a special formula. Not only are these formulas expensive, but they also taste bad to the baby.

Sleep Problems

Breastfed babies sleep less at night than formula-fed babies. Breast milk is rapidly digested, so breastfeeding babies feed more often. Keep in mind that there are benefits to frequent breastfeeding at night, both for you and your baby. (You can review the benefits of breastfeeding in chapter 1.)

Before deciding to give your baby (or yourself) a sleep remedy, consider the fact that your baby may be sleeping in an entirely normal manner for his age. Babies wake at night for many reasons—teething, a new routine, or a developmental milestone, just to name a few. It is possible that a wakeful baby is ill, so call your doctor to discuss the situation if needed. Talk to a breastfeeding helper, too. Although sleepless nights aren't much fun, there are ways to cope with what is often a temporary situation. For example, you can nap while your baby naps so you can catch up on some sleep.

Sedating your baby isn't the best answer and may be dangerous. Although breastfed babies are at a lower risk of dying from Sudden Infant Death Syndrome, the use of sedatives may interfere with this natural protection.

Remedies for Common Health Conditions

Once you have identified a health problem, it's time to think about the best ways to help your baby. Do no more than you have to, as children respond very well to the mildest treatments. (Why use an ax to cut butter?) Consider the following list of actions and remedies, which are ordered from the mildest to the most aggressive.

1. Consider remedial actions first. Skin-to-skin contact with your baby may calm him down or wake him up, depending on what is needed. Carrying your baby in a sling that wraps around your chest may lessen his crying time and help him to sleep better at night. Giving your child a massage and bathing together are other ways to get skin-to-skin contact. These simple measures can help your baby if he isn't feeling well. Whether your child has a cold, is teething, or is ill in the hospital, give him the gift of your presence. Simple human touch is a basic and powerful healing force.

Don't overlook the little things you can do to make your child feel better. Some remedial actions are so basic that they may be overlooked in the rush to treat with drugs. A tepid sponge bath can bring a high fever down quicker than a dose of Tylenol, for example. (Just don't let your baby get chilled and start shivering.) Of course, if your baby has a really high fever, you need to call the doctor regardless of what remedies you're using, as a serious infection may be the cause. Don't avoid medical care at the cost of your child's health.

2. If you want to give your child an herbal remedy, take it yourself instead of feeding it to your baby. In our culture, we often assume that treating an illness means "taking something" such as a prescription drug or an over-the-counter medication. So, when it comes to our children, our first impulse is to have them take something. Nursing mothers have another option, however. You can take an herbal remedy, and your baby may be helped by what goes through your milk.

Note that this isn't the case with drugs and medications. For example, you can't take an antibiotic to help your baby heal from an infection. But when it comes to certain herbal remedies, their helpful properties will pass through your milk to your baby. For example, you could take echinacea to help your baby heal more quickly from a cold. The echinacea boosts your immune system, and your body is stimulated to produce more infection-fighting cells in your breast milk, which help your baby to recover from his illness. Because trying to feed nasty-tasting echinacea to a baby is a daunting task, it's easier—and still effective—to simply take it yourself. Similarly, garlic is a great infection-fighter, but feeding garlic (particularly fresh garlic) to a baby can be dangerous. It's much safer for you to eat the garlic; the volatile infection-fighting constituents will pass to your milk in baby-sized amounts.

Another good reason to avoid giving herbal preparations to your baby: These feedings will likely lessen the amount of breast milk your baby is willing to take. Infants take only about 2 oz. of breast milk per feeding, so if you're also giving your baby teaspoons of herbal tea, he will quickly get full and may resist nursing. When a baby is ill, it is important to maximize his intake of breast milk, which is filled with infection-fighting antibodies.

In many cultures around the world, nursing mothers treat colic by taking fragrant herbs—most notably catnip, fennel, dill, and anise—in the form of teas. Their breastfeeding babies benefit from these time-tested remedies. The volatile, fragrant parts of these plants easily pass into breast milk and, even in tiny amounts, can help soothe a baby's digestive system. (See the discussion of colic at the end of this chapter.)

Note that some of these herbs are known to increase milk supply. When the milk is abundant and comes out too fast, your baby may react. Be aware of this side effect in certain herbs. For more information on herbal side effects, see chapter 7 and appendix C.

3. As a last resort, consider feeding an herbal remedy directly to your child. Babies younger than six months who are exclusively breastfeeding shouldn't be given anything other than breast milk without good reason, as this introduces new risks. Whether you're considering baby formula, other liquids, solid foods, herbal medicines, or drugs, always ask: "Is

there a better choice here, another way to address the problem?" Children older than six months who are eating a wide variety of foods don't face a unique allergic risk from herbs; however, it is always wise to introduce potentially allergenic foods or herbs carefully.

There may be times when feeding an herbal medicine directly to your child is the best course of action. In such cases, it is important to investigate the proper way to give the remedy. Using a bottle or a pacifier dispenser may confuse your baby if he is still learning to feed at the breast. Try a spoon, a soft feeding cup, or a medicine dropper instead. Be sure you know how to safely administer fluids to a young baby. (Ask your doctor, a nurse, or a lactation specialist.)

Rarely is there only one herb or herbal product to choose from, so comparing your options is essential. Below are some basic guidelines for using herbal remedies with children. It's best to seek expert assistance from a knowledgeable herbalist, in addition to discussing your treatment choices with your child's pediatrician.

- Use the most specific and simple herbal preparation possible. Remedies that are known to work well for a specific condition will, in general, require the smallest material dose and get the best and quickest response. It's easier to trace an allergic reaction when a simple (one herb) remedy has been tried. Herbal expert Rosemary Gladstar suggests testing for sensitivity by applying a small amount of an infusion (tea) to the skin and waiting twenty-four hours before giving it by mouth. Any sign of irritation may indicate sensitivity.

- Seek guidance to determine the appropriate dose. Children are very sensitive, and therefore very responsive, to herbs. Only the gentlest herbs are needed. The dose is always determined by the child's weight. (This is true whether you're using herbs or drugs.) Much care is needed to determine a safe dose with infants whose organs may be less able to metabolize chemicals. Always use the smallest dose that works, for the shortest time possible. With infants under a year or so, seek guidance from an herbalist before administering any herbal remedy on your own.

Applying herbs externally generally ensures that your child receives a very small dose. Yet, not all external applications of herbs, herbal preparations, or essential oils are suitable for infants and small children. You can read more about external applications later in this chapter. Homeopathic remedies contain the smallest material doses of herbs and may be more suitable than other forms for infants and children. (See appendix A for Miranda Castro's book on using homeopathics with infants.)

Be aware that long-term use of any remedy may mask serious problems. If there is no improvement in your child after a few days, take him to the doctor.

• Keep your child's physician in the loop. This is vital whenever a child has a serious illness or is taking any OTC or prescription medications. Although physicians may not often use herbs with sick children, parents certainly do. A recent survey of children with cancer showed that most of the parents were using herbs and nutritional supplements to complement their child's conventional care. Other surveys have found that children with chronic or serious illnesses are likely to be given herbs or other dietary supplements by their parents, yet few doctors specifically ask about such use. As a nursing mother, it's up to you to inform your child's healthcare providers about the herbs or other complementary therapies you're using with your child.

Some herbs are especially suited for use with babies and young children, having fewer and milder adverse effects when compared to over-the-counter or prescription medications. When choosing an herb over a drug, be sure you understand what the drug alternative is, as well as how its particular risks and benefits compare to those of the chosen herb. When using herbs in addition to conventional medicines, be sure you know how this will affect your baby's care. Drug-herb interactions are not well understood, particularly in children. Again, keep your child's pediatrician informed about any herbal therapies you are giving to your child, especially when other drugs are also being used. Don't wait for the doctor to ask if you're giving herbs or medications to your child. Instead, offer the information on your own.

Some physicians may not be comfortable with giving any herbs to children. Listen to their concerns as these doctors may have information you don't. But don't hesitate to share your own herbal research with the doctors. Remember that your relationship with your child's healthcare providers is a partnership.

Using Herbs Safely and Effectively

In our grandmothers' day, it may have seemed safe and perfectly acceptable to offer herbs and other healing plants to babies, but this is no longer the case. Today, we are facing an epidemic of food allergies (to peanuts and wheat, for example) and conditions of hypersensitivity (such as asthma and eczema). We know that these problems are best avoided by feeding only breast milk to babies in the first six months of life. Most of us wouldn't dream of feeding orange juice to a two-month-old, so what makes us assume that other plants are any safer?

Below you'll find a list of actions to take for a colicky baby. I provide this example for two reasons: (1) to show that some treatments are safer and more effective than others and (2) to offer a model for approaching other health problems your child might have.

Colic can make the early weeks and months of life miserable for both mother and baby. Colic often disappears around four months of age, well before most experts advise feeding an infant anything but breast milk. Therefore, this condition needs special scrutiny when it comes to considering safe options for treatment. And because a colicky baby is in misery, his mother and father may be desperate to do something—anything—to make the crying stop.

Typical suggestions for colic usually focus on feeding something to the baby: simethicone drops, for example, or fennel tea. Good old gripewater, still sold in Canada and in other British Commonwealth nations, contains carminative (gas-relieving) herbs and, in its original formula, alcohol. (The alcohol content alone may explain why this stuff works to quiet the baby.) Clearly, this remedy may not be the best choice in the eyes of some. And while many of the colic herbs do indeed help calm digestion, they may also cause allergy. Anise and fennel, for example, contain small amounts of the allergen trans-anethole.

So, what is a mother to do? There are lots of things to try, all safer than feeding colic herbs to your baby. Here are some possible actions and remedies:

- Talk to your breastfeeding helpers. La Leche League Leaders in particular are familiar with techniques to soothe a baby suffering from colic. There are quite a few "tricks" suggested in *The Womanly Art of Breastfeeding* or in the many books by Dr. William Sears. Talking with a La Leche Leader or another nursing mother who knows how colic can turn your life upside down can be a big help. Just having someone listen to you can be a great stress reliever.

- Try the "colic hold." Lay your child on his belly across your forearm, with your hand supporting his chest, his head slightly higher than his feet. This position can have instantaneous results for some babies.

- Take a warm bath together. The skin-to-skin contact and soothing waters can bring relief to your child.

- Try homeopathics, which may be a safer option than herbs. There are specific homeopathic remedies for colic that work quickly. A number of companies produce ready-made (and essentially risk-free) remedies.

- Give your baby a warm bath with chamomile or lavender flower infusions. Add only enough of the tea to barely color the water. (Strain out the plant matter.)

- Wrap your baby in something soothing. Try a towel soaked in warm chamomile or lavender flower tea, and gently wrap it around your baby's abdomen. Make sure the wrap isn't too hot. A drop or two of the essential oils in hot water can substitute for an infusion.

- Give your baby a gentle abdominal massage. Rub his abdomen with circular motions around the umbilicus, using olive or almond oil. Whether you're massaging his belly or rubbing his back, rhythmic skin massage can help your baby relax.

- Add soothing essential oils to your baby's massage oil. Use caraway or chamomile essential oil diluted in olive or almond oil (a ratio of 10 percent essential oil to 90 percent olive or almond oil).

- Take a colic tea yourself. Anise, fennel, caraway, cumin, and dill seed teas can help your breastfeeding baby. Use 1 teaspoon of crushed seeds with boiling water to make 6 oz. of tea (cover to steep). Note, though, that these seeds may increase your milk supply. Catnip and chamomile teas are also effective with colic and may not increase your milk supply as much as the seeds. You may need to drink several cups of tea per day to help your baby.

- Add probiotics such as yogurt, kefir, or lactobacillus capsules to your diet. These supplements may greatly improve your baby's condition if the colic is caused by substances passing into your milk. Probiotics will improve the integrity and function of your gastrointestinal tract, lessening the amount of allergens and other irritating substances that leak into your bloodstream and enter your breast milk. Ask your doctor or a naturopath about taking digestive enzyme capsules with your meals. The supplementary enzymes can help break down proteins more completely, eliminating those that may provoke your baby's colic.

- Avoiding certain foods is widely thought to prevent or help treat colic. Mothers are often advised to avoid onion, garlic, hot peppers, and cabbage, although many women have found that eating these foods does not make their babies colicky. A baby can become colicky after his mother eats a certain food, but this trigger food may vary from mother to mother. For some, it may be green beans or tomatoes. For others, brewer's yeast, vitamins with iron or fluoride, or artificial sweeteners. Mothers who smoke or who drink large amounts of caffeine tend to have colicky babies. If you can eliminate trigger foods and substances from your diet, you should see positive results within a day or so, although the full effect may not be apparent for a week or two.

- As a last resort, feed your baby colic tea. Colic teas can work very quickly, but they should be considered only in the most desperate situations, when you really need your baby to stop crying NOW in order to keep your sanity. There are good reasons for not trying this method first. Besides being potentially allergenic, teas and similar preparations can quickly fill up an infant's stomach, which means the baby will take less breast milk. If you must feed your baby herbal teas, use an eyedropper or a spoon instead of a bottle. But don't rely on herbs as your mainstay of colic treatment. Start with the safer ways of giving herbal remedies, as they have a good chance of working.

External Use of Herbs

Many mothers want to use herbal products on their baby's skin for skin care, soothing baths, or massage, or they want to use herbs in vaporizers and "sleep pillows." But babies can be extremely sensitive to anything that comes in contact with their skin or lungs, so it's important to use caution.

The body can absorb very small amounts of many substances applied to the skin. This may be especially true for babies and small children, whose skin is thin, soft, and tender. If you want to use essential oils on

Homemade Baby Formula: A Bad Idea

Humans have experimented with substitutes for human breast milk since the beginning of time. It wasn't until the mid-twentieth century that a fairly decent substitute for breast milk was developed and marketed (decent in that it saved more babies than it killed). When I was a child, buying ready-made formula was unheard of in farm families. People were given a recipe to make formula at home: canned milk, corn syrup, and, if your doctor was an advanced thinker, multivitamin drops. Unfortunately, I grew up on some version of this stuff, as did many other baby boomers. In the late sixties, homemade baby formula still seemed the way to go, since many young people believed that the formula companies were "evil" and any concoction made with health food was good.

There are a lot of different recipes for homemade baby formula, including some that use soymilk and some that use goat's milk. Well-meaning herbalists sometimes suggest putting nature-based vitamin and mineral supplements into homemade baby formulas. But these recipes are never a good substitute for commercial baby formula, and certainly not for breast milk; they aren't even safe for infants. For example, plain soymilk lacks iodine and can therefore cause thyroid problems in babies who drink it. Because ingesting too much or too little iodine presents major health risks for babies, companies that make baby formula carefully control the amount of iodine they add to their products. This cannot be safely done at home.

Growing babies need vitamins and minerals in specific amounts and can easily become deficient or overloaded. Babies also have specific protein and water requirements. There are cases where infants have died as a result of being given baby formula that was overdiluted to make it last longer. Babies can't adapt to poor nutrition the way that older children and adults can. Formula companies spend vast amounts of money and time trying to mimic the unique properties of breast milk, and we really can't expect to duplicate their efforts in our own kitchens. If, for whatever reason, you cannot give your baby breast milk during his first year, do not give him homemade formula. Commercial baby formula is the

your child, you must first dilute them—often more than you would dilute them for an adult. (Read more about essential oils in chapter 4.) Always research a concentrated product before using it on your baby's skin.

On the other hand, this skin sensitivity means that the gentlest herbs can do wonders for babies, even when applied externally. External applications are sometimes an effective alternative to feeding an herbal remedy to a baby.

It makes sense to avoid potentially toxic, irritating, or allergenic herbs—even on intact, or unbroken, skin. Babies are much more likely to react to allergens or irritants than adults are. If you use a plant that is known to cause allergic reactions, be cautious. Try a patch test first. To do this, apply a weak solution of the herb to a small area of your baby's skin and check for a reaction after twenty-four hours.

Dangerous Practices

It may seem obvious, but toxic herbs should be completely avoided. Always use gentle, nontoxic herbs. Comfrey, for example, is frequently included in skin care products and herbal recipes, yet this herb sometimes contains a toxic alkaloid that is considered dangerous for use during breastfeeding or with young children. In Germany, it is forbidden to sell any comfrey product that contains more than 1 part per million of the toxic alkaloid. Even the external use of comfrey is restricted. Do not use comfrey on your child. Instead, use calendula petals or other wound healers that are more baby-friendly.

Some strong-smelling essential oils—peppermint, eucalyptus, tea tree, neroli, and camphor—require special precautions around small children. Placing these essential oils on or near your baby's face, particularly on or near his nose, can cause breathing problems. There have been several cases where parents put products made from peppermint oil in their infant's nose, and, almost immediately, the baby stopped breathing. It is also important to avoid using these oils on your chest, so your baby won't be affected when nursing. However, some of these oils (eucalyptus oil, for example) can be used safely in room vaporizers.

Nutritional Supplements

Not so long ago, pediatricians routinely directed mothers to give their breastfed babies iron, vitamin, and fluoride supplements. In recent years, such supplements have been viewed with more caution and are no longer routinely suggested. Pediatricians with expertise in lactation have long considered such supplements as unnecessary and possibly risky (iron, for example).

The current controversy over vitamin D typifies how routine practices have waxed and waned over the years. Most breastfed babies do not need vitamin D supplements. If your healthcare provider suggests supplementing your baby's diet with vitamin D, consider whether it is truly necessary. Lighter-skinned babies need only a few minutes of sunlight on their faces daily to make sufficient vitamin D. On the other hand, if you don't take your baby out in the sun at all or if you cover him in clothing or apply strong sunscreen from head to toe when he does go out, he may need a vitamin D supplement. Likewise, if he has more deeply pigmented skin (which slows vitamin D formation), you may also need to give him a vitamin D supplement. In the absence of these factors, there may be little need for vitamin D supplements.

Do not try to supplement your own diet with vitamin D, as the amount required to increase vitamin D levels in breast milk would be toxic for you. Ask your lactation helper for current information on this issue.

Herbal Tonics and Health Drinks

Tonic supplements are widely used around the world, typically as teas, to strengthen babies against potential problems. However, babies who are given tonic teas have poorer health compared to babies who are not given tonic teas and who are exclusively breastfed instead. It cannot be repeated enough: Most exclusively breastfed babies do not need vitamin, mineral, or tonic supplements. These products can actually cause harm. In the early months of your baby's life, 100 percent breast milk is best.

Babies older than one year are able to eat most solid foods, and most can tolerate cow's milk as well. This age is considered safe for serving homemade health drinks, and many toddlers seem to enjoy them. If you want to improve your toddler's nutrition or if he is a very picky eater, health drinks are a reasonable option. You can try drinks made with animal milk (goat or sheep) or vegetable protein milk (soy, rice, or oat). Some moms add a little bit of barley or alfalfa juice powder (don't use too much, as the dark color repels toddlers), fruit, or fruit concentrates to help make the drink tasty. Ready-to-mix nutritional products aimed at children are increasingly common on store shelves. Watch out, however, for products high in sugar or that contain adult-sized doses of vitamins or minerals.

Where to Go for More Information

A number of good herbal books offer information on the use of herbs with children. (See appendix A.) Look for comprehensive books written by Master Herbalists. Rosemary Gladstar's *Herbal Remedies for Children's Health* is a good starting point. The author makes clear that herbal remedies should be given to mothers of breastfed babies rather than to the babies themselves, and she includes herbal suggestions for routine skin care and other types of preventive care. Some of her recipes, however, include comfrey, which I recommend avoiding, especially with a small baby. Aviva Romm's book *Naturally Healthy Babies and Children* features a comprehensive discussion about incorporating herbs into the care of children (although, again, comfrey is sometimes suggested for skin care). Overall, Romm's book includes a wealth of suggestions, and its foreword was written by breastfeeding-friendly pediatrician Dr. William Sears. If you're looking for a good homeopathic book, try Miranda Castro's classic *Homeopathy for Pregnancy, Birth and Your Baby's First Year.*

❦ ❦ ❦

When your baby is sick, special care is required. No matter what remedies you may use or which alternative healthcare practitioners you see, your child's doctor should be consulted if a problem persists or worsens or new symptoms appear. When you are ill, the doctor is but a phone call away; but a sick child depends on you to make that call for him. A consultation with your child's doctor is essential. Whatever treatments you and your doctor decide upon rarely need to interfere with breastfeeding. Continuing to breastfeed ensures that your child will get the healthy benefits that only your milk can provide.

$\mathscr{W}$eaning and the Return to Fertility

The word *weaning* means different things to different people. To some, it is an event; to others, it is a process. If you think about it, your child is weaning from the moment he starts eating table foods. It is then that he moves away from exclusive breastfeeding toward the time when he no longer receives even a smidgen of breast milk at bedtime. A child who no longer takes any breast milk is weaned.

Weaning can happen unexpectedly, or it can be carefully planned. Or, it may simply occur as it is an inevitable outcome of a child's development. For some, weaning happens all at once; for others, it occurs over a number of years. How and when weaning happens is up to you or your child (whoever takes the lead). But even if you do nothing to stop breastfeeding, weaning happens all the same.

As a nursing mother, you may often be asked, "When are you going to stop breastfeeding?" Like many other aspects of motherhood, everyone seems to have an opinion about weaning. You may find that the people around you—family, friends, and breastfeeding helpers—greatly

Weaning for "Health Reasons"

Perhaps you or your child has a health issue that your doctor feels is "caused by breastfeeding" or "can't be treated unless you wean." It is imperative to gather more information before accepting this advice as fact. In almost all circumstances, there are ways to preserve the breastfeeding relationship. Seek more information from a breastfeeding specialist.

influence your thoughts about weaning. It certainly is a ripe topic of discussion when nursing mothers get together! One thing is clear: The issue of weaning is as emotional and complex as the topic of breastfeeding itself. There are many ways to go about weaning, and they depend on a number of factors: your needs, your child's needs, your values and beliefs, your family, and your personal feelings.

With so many things to consider, where do you begin? It helps to talk to an experienced breastfeeding helper, as well as other mothers who have been through weaning. These women can help you understand the various methods for weaning a child and their possible outcomes.

There are many articles and books for mothers who are thinking about weaning. One book in particular stands out as a "must read": *How Weaning Happens* by Diane Bengston, published by La Leche League International (see appendix A). This book covers the whole territory of weaning, always underscoring the important La Leche League principle that, whenever possible, weaning should occur gradually, with love. If you can gradually reduce nursing while increasing the level of emotional support, care, and attention that you bestow on your child, both you and your child will experience immeasurable benefits.

Family and Personal Issues

For some mothers, weaning becomes an issue for the baby's father, particularly if he feels that breastfeeding is interfering with his relationship with his wife or child. If you find yourself in this situation, this is a good time to connect with your breastfeeding supporters (see chapter 2). You may want to attend La Leche League meetings to talk with other mothers who can help you sort out the emotional issues surrounding this critical topic. Some families are able to compromise with partial weaning (continuing breastfeeding but not at certain times or places).

Perhaps you need to go back to work, and you aren't sure whether you can manage breastfeeding and working at the same time. Talk to other working mothers who are breastfeeding so you can get their input. Fortunately, things are changing in the workplace as more employers recognize the value of helping their employees continue breastfeeding. There are challenges for nursing mothers who work, but there are also resources and solutions for problems. Many mothers feel that the physical and emotional benefits of breastfeeding outweigh the challenges. Others decide that partial weaning is necessary. Delaying your return to work or working only part-time can reduce the need to pump at work, if this option doesn't seem possible for you. Look into all your options before deciding to wean.

Temporary weaning is a different situation. You may be advised to wean temporarily if you need to use a particular medication, for example. Be assured, however, that very few medications require the temporary disruption of breastfeeding. It's essential to talk to a lactation specialist who has access to the latest information on medications and can help guide your choices.

If you must disrupt breastfeeding in order to take a medication you really need, all is not lost. If you have some lead time, you may be able to pump and store enough breast milk to supply your baby during the temporary weaning period. Continue to pump (and dump the milk) during the time that your baby can't nurse, so you can maintain your milk supply. This way, there will be breast milk ready for your baby once the medication is gone from your body.

Many babies who stop breastfeeding temporarily will immediately start nursing at the breast again, as if nothing had happened. Others need persistent coaching to get back to the breast. Although it's true that some babies won't nurse again after a temporary disruption, never say never. See what your baby will do at the breast before assuming that he won't nurse; you never know until you try. And keep on trying— gently. Even weeks of refusal can end with the baby suddenly latching on and breastfeeding. Consult with your breastfeeding helpers. They can guide you to a good pump and offer suggestions for getting your baby back to the breast. They can also provide the emotional support to get you through, no matter how things end.

Some nursing mothers are told to wean in preparation for breast surgery. If you are advised to wean before or after breast surgery, investigate your options. Not all surgeons are familiar with the lactating breast, and much depends on the type of surgery—many conditions don't require weaning. With good information, the surgeon may be able to operate in a way that minimizes the impact on breastfeeding. If your situation requires weaning, you may be able to slow or stop milk production on the affected breast (simply by not offering that breast to

Losing Your Baby

The tragedy of losing a baby can be compounded when milk and engorgement adds to a mother's heavy burden of grief. Some mothers choose to pump their milk and donate it to a milk bank, finding some solace in knowing that their milk is going to help others in need. Other mothers find this option unbearable and want to stop the milk as quickly as possible. This is an extremely personal decision, and mothers should reach out to breastfeeding helpers who will understand and assist them, no matter what they decide to do.

your baby), yet continue to nurse with the other breast. Not all surgeons will think of this option, so be sure to bring it up. Many babies nurse quite well on one breast, as surely as twins can nurse successfully on two breasts. This situation may be temporary or permanent. Again, a breast-feeding helper can guide you through this process.

About Weaning

Entire books have been written on weaning, and I encourage you to look into a few of them before you actually begin to wean your child. This chapter doesn't describe all of the various methods available. Instead, it focuses on how herbs can be used safely during weaning. It also discusses fertility, which, for some women, returns only after weaning.

If you're able to take a gradual approach to weaning, you don't need to do anything in particular to stay comfortable while your breasts slow the production of milk. A gradual weaning process should prevent engorgement. However, if you do experience painful engorgement, don't allow it to continue. The pain means you must, by whatever means, remove some milk from your breasts. You may need to take weaning more slowly, if possible. (For information on engorgement, see chapter 8.) Keep in mind that every woman is different. Some may be able to wean quickly without engorgement; others may need to take more time.

If you must wean abruptly, do so safely, because engorgement is painful and can damage the breasts. Engorgement also puts you at risk for mastitis. (Read about mastitis in chapter 8.) Here are the current recommendations for rapidly drying up milk:

- Wear a snug-fitting bra (but not so tight as to bind). The bra should offer uniform counter-resistance to the engorgement. You may need a bigger bra size than before.

- Binding the breasts is not recommended. It doesn't speed the weaning process, and putting pressure on the breasts can cause pain, plugged ducts, mastitis, and abscesses.

- Do not restrict your fluids, as this won't help. Continue to drink enough to adequately quench your thirst. Limiting your salt intake may help reduce water retention.

- If engorgement becomes uncomfortable or painful, or if leaking of milk occurs, you can gently express some milk, as often as needed. Sometimes, removing only a few drops is all that is necessary for relief. Just don't completely empty the breasts, as this will restimulate your milk supply. The goal is to express just enough milk to relieve your discomfort and prevent plugged ducts and mastitis. Note: Women who choose to bottle feed after birth are often told not to express any milk. Your situation is different, however. As a mother who has been breastfeeding, you will probably need to express some milk to prevent pain and severe engorgement.

- Express some milk at night so you don't wake up in the morning with rock-hard, painful breasts. As long as only small amounts of milk are removed, your milk supply will continue to decrease, and so will your need to remove milk for comfort.

- You can place cabbage leaves on both breasts to help reduce your milk supply more quickly. Most women find that the leaves are more comfortable than ice packs, and they work about as well (no better and no worse). You may need to use the leaves for several days. (For details, see chapter 8.)

- Wear nursing pads to absorb any milk that leaks. Change the pads as often as needed.

- Try to avoid nipple stimulation during this time, but don't avoid cuddling your baby. He will need lots of extra love and attention from you during the time it takes to wean.

- If you are very uncomfortable, you may need to take a pain reliever; anti-inflammatory painkillers (such as ibuprofen) or anti-inflammatory herbal remedies can help. See chapter 8 for more information.

- Consider using sage, parsley, and peppermint. These herbs have long been used to dry up milk supply. See the discussion below. Chapter 8 also includes information on how these herbs may affect milk production.

At one time, certain medications were widely used to suppress milk production, and the most notorious of these was bromocriptine (also known as Parlodel). This drug is no longer recommended because it (1) presents a risk of stroke and (2) has only a temporary effect—the milk supply will rebound once the mother has discontinued use of the drug. If your doctor prescribes this drug to suppress lactation, be sure to discuss the risks and then seek a second opinion. Newer medications are available, but you'll need to look carefully at the pros and cons of each.

You may feel that over-the-counter medications are a better option than prescription drugs. Over-the-counter medications containing pseudoephedrine and certain antihistamines have been found to slow or stop milk production. Talk to a lactation specialist to learn more about these options.

Weaning Herbs

Certain herbs, called antigalactogogues, have been found to lower milk supply. For this reason, they may be useful if you need to quickly lower your supply or stop milk production altogether. You may need to take them for quite a while; otherwise, a well-established milk supply may rebound, leaving you engorged again. Although there are no scientific studies regarding the use of these herbs in slowing or stopping milk production, traditional and anecdotal evidence suggests that they might be useful for many women. Chapter 7 includes detailed information on the antigalactogogue herbs peppermint, parsley, and sage, which are sometimes used in combination with cabbage leaves and ice.

In general, larger quantities of weaning herbs are used to dry up a milk supply, and smaller quantities to slow it down. Sage is probably the most active in lowering supply and has long been known as the herb of choice for active weaning. You need to be careful with sage, however. Overdose reactions (rapid heart rate, hot flashes, convulsions, dizziness) can occur if 15 or more grams of sage are taken at one time. Stick to the doses described in chapter 7. Another word of caution: Tincture and liquid extract forms of sage may vary in concentration and cannot be safely used in high doses for long periods of time. (Do not use for more than a week.) Sage essential oil is toxic when taken internally and should be avoided. As engorgement decreases, reduce the amount of sage you are using. Consider switching to peppermint oil or parsley.

You may want to use homeopathic preparations for weaning. Herbalist Mechell Turner, IBCLC, suggests homeopathic *Lac caninum* to prevent engorgement. See her web site at www.birthandbreastfeeding.com for dose suggestions, or ask a homeopathic practitioner for more information.

In rapid weaning situations, you should be in contact with a lactation specialist who can help you adjust herb dosages depending on your individual needs. Women vary in how they respond to herbal remedies. Some women can lower their milk supply with small doses of anti-galactogogue herbs (a couple cups of peppermint tea, for example). Other women find that large doses of these herbs hardly affect their milk supply at all. Some wise women have suggested that unless the mother is definite about her decision to wean, no amount of herbs will help her. Perhaps this is true as well. If you're unsure about whether you and your child are truly ready to wean, reach out to your breastfeeding supporters. Talk with them about your concerns.

What to Expect after Weaning

After weaning has occurred, it takes about two weeks for the breast to return to a nonlactating state. You may continue to produce a little milk for quite a long time after weaning, though. This is normal. Occasionally, milk in the breasts during the months or years after weaning may indicate a medical problem, so it may be wise to consult with your doctor. Yet, many healthy women who nursed for extended periods of time continue to have milk in their breasts long after weaning has taken place. I know of one woman who got used to having a wet blouse whenever she held a new niece or nephew for the first time! This went on many years after her last child had weaned.

Fertility and Your Menstrual Cycle

It has long been known that breastfeeding is a cheap, safe, and effective means of birth control, and science has confirmed this traditional knowledge. Intensive research of nursing mothers has resulted in the Lactation Amenorrhea Method (LAM) of contraception. This method is easily learned and gives mothers a degree of control over their fertility. Mothers who (1) are exclusively breastfeeding, with no use of pacifiers or bottles, (2) have babies ages six months or younger, and (3) haven't yet had their menstrual cycle return are 98 percent unlikely to become pregnant in the first six months after birth. In the first six months especially, the return to fertility is usually marked with a menstrual period before ovulation occurs. After six months, women who have not had a period may continue to be infertile, but the risk of pregnancy rises. LAM is taught to women throughout the world as a safe, reliable alternative to hormonal birth control methods.

In La Leche League's book *The Womanly Art of Breastfeeding,* Dr. Herbert Ratner says: "It is the baby's sucking that controls the mother's ovulation. The more the baby has a need to suck, the less ready he is to be displaced by another. The less the baby has a need to suck, the more ready and able he is to cope with a new brother or sister."[11] Mothers who have babies who want to nurse frequently, day or night, often find that their menstrual periods may not return for well over a year, or even two years. This can be a good or bad thing, depending on whether the mother wishes to become pregnant again.

For more information on LAM, see the following section on preventing pregnancy. Additional resources are listed in appendices A and B.

Preventing Pregnancy

New mothers become fertile again at varying lengths of time after giving birth. For some, any amount of breastfeeding prevents pregnancy. Others get their menstrual periods once again within three months of their baby's birth, even if they're breastfeeding exclusively and frequently. Regularly recurring periods usually indicate the return of fertility, a time when decisions about birth control need to be made.

According to LAM, there is little reason to use a form of synthetic hormonal birth control for the first six months after your child is born, as long as the mother exclusively breastfeeds her baby, with no use of pacifiers or bottles, and hasn't yet had her menstrual cycle. LAM can always be combined with barrier methods of birth control, such as condoms or a diaphragm, for additional reassurance. After the return of regular menstrual periods, look for birth control that doesn't contain estrogen, as synthetic estrogen is associated with decreased milk supply. Agents containing only progesterone haven't been shown to change milk supply, but they're still being studied to determine their safety for the breastfeeding mother and child. Some healthcare professionals and lactation specialists conservatively suggest avoiding any synthetic hormones while nursing, though no evidence has, as yet, shown that these agents will harm a breastfeeding baby.

For more detailed information on fertility and breastfeeding, you may want to read Sheila Kippley's *Breastfeeding and Natural Child Spacing* and Merryl Winstein's *Your Fertility Signals*. Both books are listed in appendix A. La Leche League groups often have these books in their libraries.

Since the time of antiquity, herbal authors have recorded the ways in which plants affect fertility. The ancient physicians of Greece and Rome wrote detailed accounts of plants that were specifically used to prevent conception or to end a pregnancy. Midwives were the experts on the use of such agents, which were always a matter of societal debate and regulation. (For a full history, read *Eve's Herbs* by John Riddle, which is listed in appendix A.) Herbs known today as emmenagogues (or those that bring on delayed menstrual periods) were often used with the intent to induce an abortion during the first trimester. It was widely understood that the herbs and activities the midwives warned mothers against during pregnancy were often used to end a pregnancy.

While not all herbs that work to end a pregnancy are toxic, some definitely are; they work by poisoning the fetus. These toxic plants should be avoided at all costs, as they can also endanger the mother's life. The dose required to end a pregnancy is often enough to be toxic for an adult. Pennyroyal oil is probably the most infamous of these herbs. A number of women have died after taking the essential oil to induce abortion. Seek expert herbalist and medical guidance before you consider ending a pregnancy by herbal means.

Many herbs have been used since antiquity to reduce fertility by preventing conception. Unlike some abortifacient herbs, they are non-toxic and probably work through hormonal influences. A remarkable number of such herbs are also traditionally used to increase milk supply. Some are known to increase prolactin levels and thus indirectly suppress ovulation. This action is akin to a mother nursing frequently to ensure that ovulation remains suppressed.

Certain herbs, such as wild carrot seed and blessed thistle, have traditionally been used to prevent conception. Scientific studies indicate that these herbs may indeed have a contraceptive effect, and scientists plan to study them further. As yet, however, there is little scientific information on how effective these plants are as contraceptives. Most of what we know comes through the traditional knowledge of herbalist midwives.

Because synthetic hormone methods of birth control have seen such widespread acceptance around the world, herbal studies have been seriously neglected. This may change now that the risks associated with synthetic hormones are becoming more apparent to women and their doctors. Be sure to seek expert herbalist assistance if you wish to explore herbal contraceptives as a birth control option. While many herbalists consider herbs safer than synthetic hormones, if contraception is really important to you, you may want to hedge your bets by using a combination of approaches, instead of just one, to prevent conception. (For more on this topic, see appendix A for books by Sheila Kippley and Susun Weed and appendix B for contact information for the Couple to Couple League.)

It may come as a surprise to you to learn that a number of foods are suspected of reducing fertility. For example, many legumes (members of the pea family) have traditionally been used to reduce fertility, and a few scientific studies confirm this effect. According to one study on human subjects, eating large quantities of cooked dried peas every day significantly lessened the chance of conceiving. These findings should not concern you unless you eat the same foods day in and day out. It is always wise to eat a wide variety of plant foods, and not rely on just a few while trying to become pregnant.

Increasing Fertility

Many mothers choose to wean in order to increase fertility if they've been unable to get pregnant while breastfeeding. In the case of women who are seeking help from a fertility clinic, the doctors often will not authorize treatment until breastfeeding has stopped, because they fear that the powerful synthetic hormones that are used in fertility treatments may harm a nursing child. And because nursing is known to affect fertility, they feel that breastfeeding should end before medical fertility treatments begin. Indeed, some women just can't get pregnant as long as their child is nursing, even if he nurses only at bedtime.

If you're facing the dilemma of whether to wean your toddler in order to become pregnant again, take a little time to sort through all your options. True, you may hear that biological clock ticking and feel a sense of urgency about your situation. You may worry that you don't have time to wait for your child to wean himself. Or, you might try to start weaning gradually, only to find that your child seems distressed. Some women are understandably very uncomfortable about forcing a reluctant child to wean. Yet, fertility is already decreased by the time a woman reaches her mid-thirties—your window of opportunity may, in fact, be coming to a close. Contact a lactation specialist for more information about your particular situation and what your best course of action may be.

Depending on your situation, there is an herb for infertility that may be preferable even to partial weaning. Chasteberry, also known as vitex, has been used for centuries to normalize menstrual periods. In Germany, modern-day studies have shown chasteberry to be effective for women who have scanty, infrequent periods (and suffer from PMS and infertility as well). Not only did the length of the women's periods become more normal, but many of the women who were previously infertile became pregnant after taking the herb. In fact, chasteberry is used as a first-line fertility treatment by many German physicians, being a safer alternative to conventional hormone treatments. The plant has no evidence of toxicity, and side effects (allergic rash, headaches, nausea) are very rare.

Mothers who use chasteberry to speed a return to fertility may see their milk supply decrease. But once they become pregnant, their milk supply will decrease anyway. Nursing toddlers seem to work through this loss pretty well. They can see for themselves that there is very little milk. Some will continue nursing for comfort, while others will stop all together. And some give up nursing only until the milk returns after birth, and then they want to nurse again.

German herb experts currently recommend that nursing mothers avoid chasteberry, because they fear it may lower milk supply, not because it presents a danger to the child. Lab studies show that high doses of chasteberry reduce prolactin and milk production in rats. Yet, chasteberry has traditionally been used to increase milk supply, and some herbalists continue to use it as a galactogogue. Others say that if used for too long, chasteberry causes the milk supply to dwindle. The dose and the length of time it is used may determine its effect; however, modern studies of breastfeeding women have not been done to confirm this. What we do know from older studies is that nursing mothers who used chasteberry for longer than two weeks had their periods return early. You can look in appendix C for a profile on chasteberry. If you're interested in using this herb, ask a lactation specialist and your healthcare provider for guidance.

As a general rule, when hoping to become pregnant, eat a varied diet. Some foods can help your chances of becoming pregnant, while others may hurt them. Unfortunately, there isn't enough information available to specify which foods may help or hurt. Rather than worry, simply eat a varied diet. By avoiding large doses of any one food day after day, you'll likely prevent any antifertility effects, as well as lower the risk of food allergies in your baby. Eating a varied and nutritious diet is essential if you're trying to become pregnant.

Appendix A points you to more information on using herbs for fertility. Books by Rosemary Gladstar and Susun Weed offer a variety of herbalist approaches to achieving pregnancy.

Breastfeeding during Pregnancy

If you've learned that you're pregnant and you're wondering if it's okay to continue nursing your child, talk to a lactation specialist. Nursing while pregnant has special challenges, but it isn't harmful for most pregnancies. Whatever you are feeling, whatever you have been told, it will help to talk about it and find out more about others who have been in your situation. La Leche League has over forty-five years of experience in providing information and support in this special circumstance.

Some women simply aren't comfortable breastfeeding while pregnant and decide to wean. Other women decide that nursing their child during pregnancy is both possible and beneficial. Moms may choose to "live through" the discomforts for the sake of a particularly needy toddler, as the alternative (weaning) may seem more difficult. This is not an easy choice for any nursing mother to make. It may help to read about these issues in depth so that you can explore the pros and cons and come to understand the experience of nursing while pregnant or tandem nursing (nursing a newborn and a toddler at the same time). Books and booklets on these special topics are available through La Leche League. Talking with other mothers who have faced these challenges is also helpful, and you can find support no matter what you decide to do.

Mothers who decide to continue nursing through a pregnancy often have a child who is at least a year old. But, occasionally, mothers will become pregnant when their baby is still exclusively breastfeeding or still taking breast milk as an important part of his diet. Then, somewhere near the fourth month of pregnancy, there's a big drop in milk production; this is natural and expected. Babies under a year old usually need some amount of formula supplementation at this point. Many mothers seek to maintain their milk supply despite the natural drop in the fourth month of pregnancy, but is it possible to reverse this natural course of lactation?

Very little information is available on this topic, though some women have reported limited success in increasing their milk supply with herbs while pregnant. I recommend caution when using herbs during pregnancy, particularly in the first and early second trimester. Many of the herbs used to increase milk supply (fenugreek and blessed thistle, for example) are also uterine stimulants; they may have strong enough actions to bring about a miscarriage. Because there is little information delineating which of the many uterine stimulant herbs may cause premature labor, it is wise to avoid many of them altogether.

If you feel you must use milk-increasing herbs during pregnancy, you may be safer taking herbs such as alfalfa and nettle, which have been used by many pregnant women without apparent risk. Alfalfa and nettle are traditionally used as *partus preparors*—herbs used to prepare the body for labor and delivery. At least one herb company, Motherlove, produces a milk-making remedy for the pregnant woman (see appendix B). This product may be safer for you, but check with a lactation specialist first.

Information about the safe use of herbs while pregnant is mainly traditional, and an herbalist midwife may be your most knowledgeable guide. Keep in mind that the list of plants to avoid or use with great caution is much longer for pregnancy than it is for lactation. Seek individualized help so you can make good choices. And if there are any special risks with your pregnancy, seek the counsel of a knowledgeable obstetrician as well.

Menstrual Problems

Once your menstrual periods return, they may be irregular, or they may be quite different from what they were before you had a child.

Breastfeeding influences the menstrual cycle, so the changes you're experiencing during lactation may be entirely normal. (La Leche League's *The Womanly Art of Breastfeeding* has a thorough introduction to this topic.) Some changes in the menstrual cycle, however, may not be normal and could indicate the need for medical guidance. Talk to a lactation specialist to help clarify whether you're experiencing normal changes or not.

Scanty or irregular periods while breastfeeding may be normal. As time goes on, you can expect ovulation and your menstrual flow to become more regular. (Usually, this happens over a number of monthly cycles.) Once you have started menstruating again, you may notice that if your breastfeeding child nurses more frequently (for whatever reason) or nurses longer, your periods stop or become scant. This, too, is probably normal.

Some women have heavier menstrual periods after they've had children. This may happen for a variety of reasons that aren't associated with breastfeeding. If you have concerns or questions about whether your heavier flow is normal, pay a visit to your healthcare provider.

Once your period returns, so might premenstrual syndrome (PMS), or it may develop for the first time. (Perhaps you have now entered your perimenopausal years.) Many of the herbal remedies that are useful for PMS are considered compatible with breastfeeding, particularly if your child is bigger and older. Still, it's always wise to know about the effects of any herbal remedy before taking it. For more information on herbs that may help, consult some of the many wonderful herbal books listed in appendix A. Check appendix C to see if the suggested herbs may affect your milk supply.

If you experience breast pain and bloating during your period, consider adding more essential fatty acids or fish oils to your diet. Evening primrose oil (EPO), black currant seed oil, and borage seed oil are well-known sources of essential fatty acids. Breastfeeding women have found that EPO helps to relieve the painful lumpy breasts that come with menstrual periods. Borage leaf contains very small amounts of a toxic alkaloid and is generally not recommended by herbalists for breastfeeding women. However, borage oil is free of this toxin; it is made from the seed, which does not contain toxic forms of pyrrolizidine alkaloids. Flaxseed meal or oil, or walnuts and walnut oil, may also help. Dandelion leaf is widely suggested for premenstrual water retention. It is preferred over uva-ursi, which may irritate the kidneys. Chasteberry can help relieve many premenstrual discomforts, yet it may affect your milk supply if taken in high doses for more than two weeks.

For painful cramps, one of the best natural comfort remedies is cramp bark, also known as guelder rose. A close relative, black haw, may also be helpful, though it shouldn't be used if you have a history of kidney stones. Cramp bark immediately acts to relieve menstrual cramps and the discomforts due to pelvic congestion. Typically, only small doses are needed, so a bottle of tincture can last through several menstrual cycles. Be sure to follow the manufacturer's instructions on the label carefully.

There are many herbal and nutritional approaches to lessen a heavy flow. See the women's herbal books in appendix A for a number of tried-and-true methods. One herb to avoid is dong quai, which is widely thought to increase menstrual flow. (However, it has traditionally been used throughout Asia to help mothers recover in the early postpartum.)

Many other herbs can help ease the discomforts of the menstrual cycle; this book merely scratches the surface of the world of helpful plants. If your menstrual cycle is a source of misery, it may be time to tap the wisdom of a healthcare provider. Your provider may be able to give you valuable information and suggest new treatment options.

Sometimes, a serious medical condition is at the root of severe menstrual symptoms. Ruling out a serious problem is important for your health. In the case of a serious medical condition, self-treatment isn't recommended. See a doctor to get a diagnosis and a medical perspective. She or he can help you determine which complementary or alternative therapies may be right for you. (Chapter 5 includes a full discussion of the range of healthcare options available to consumers.) Alternative providers also may have much to offer you. In fact, many women have found that working with a skilled practitioner using nutritional, herbal, and physical therapies can bring positive results. This may allow you to avoid surgery (hysterectomy) or the use of synthetic hormones.

❦ ❦ ❦

Issues of weaning, fertility, and infertility are complex, and there are many herbal approaches that may help you. In this chapter, I've touched on only a few of the herbal remedies that can be useful for menstrual problems. The women's books listed in appendix A contain the knowledge of many renowned herbalist midwives. Their collective wisdom can further guide your choices. You might also seek the care and attention of an herbalist midwife in your community—someone who can meet your unique, individual needs.

Many sources of herbal information overlook the extensive role that breastfeeding plays in fertility. In general, those remedies and actions that increase milk supply also act to suppress fertility. And the remedies and actions that promote fertility often lower milk supply. Traditional healers have long known the connection between breastfeeding and fertility that modern medical research is now confirming. Women respond differently to the forces that affect fertility and breastfeeding. And women have different emotional responses to becoming pregnant while breastfeeding, or to being unable to become pregnant while breastfeeding. Our personal responses add to the complexity of all these issues.

Whatever your situation, know that there are other women who have had a similar experience. Seek them out. You can find them at La Leche League meetings or other places where breastfeeding women gather. Other nursing mothers can be your greatest source of comfort, knowledge, guidance, and wisdom, from the moment you introduce your baby to the breast to the eventual time when weaning occurs.

ℱinal Thoughts

Knowledge of healing plants is an almost forgotten wisdom in modern society. At no other time in human history has it been such unfamiliar territory. Only in the modern era have we come to see herbs as unfamiliar, ineffective, and "risky."

During the twentieth century, modern medicine moved away from the traditional use of healing plants and began to view herbs as ineffective compared to scientifically produced drugs and medications. It is true that the herbs did not have the dramatic actions favored in the medical arts. And the new medicines were quick, reliable, and effective for many previously untreatable conditions. So, one by one, herbs were dropped from the official U.S. Pharmacopoeia, their virtues forgotten.

Interestingly, herbs were not dropped because they were dangerous. (Those few herbs that were dangerous were often purified and refined into relatively safer medicines.) Rather, most herbs, being gentler or slower acting, were simply ignored and then forgotten. These gentle herbs have now become so unfamiliar to conventional medicine that they're often thought out of ignorance to be more dangerous than drugs—especially when used with pregnant or nursing women and children. The European view is somewhat different, as herbal therapies have remained part of mainstream health care there. Indeed, because herbs can have fewer and milder side effects than conventional medications, many European doctors *prefer* to use herbs with nursing mothers and children.

Our ancestors knew both the benefits and the risks of herbal medicines and were very sophisticated in their use of herbs. Women have traditionally used herbs in all phases of reproduction: from conception to pregnancy, from childbirth to postpartum, and, of course, from breastfeeding to weaning. Fortunately, modern society is once again interested in learning what our ancestors knew about herbs. Scientific knowledge of how traditional peoples use plants (ethnobotany) and information about plants gleaned through modern scientific experimental research is leading to new treatments and approaches that may revolutionize health care. Meanwhile, lay people in Western society are already seeking out herbal medicines. And why not? There just might be gentler, more effective ways to solve health problems. And so we enter the realm of herbs.

Wise women have long understood that herbs can be powerful but gentle medicine. Mothers and children have much to gain from their wise use. Wise use is educated use. Hopefully, *The Nursing Mother's Herbal* contains the information you need to maintain your breastfeeding relationship, even as you integrate healing plants into your life.

Notes

1. AAP policy statement. "Transfer of drugs and other chemicals into human milk." *Pediatrics,* vol. 108, no. 3 (September 2001): 776–789.

2. Lawrence, Ruth, MD. "A Review of the Medical Benefits and Contraindications to Breastfeeding in the United States," *Maternal and Child Technical Information Bulletin,* Oct. 1997. U.S. Dept. of Health and Human Services, Public Health Service; Heather McLean. *Women's Experience of Breastfeeding.* Toronto: University of Toronto Press, 1990.

3. La Leche League International. *The Womanly Art of Breastfeeding.* 6th ed. Schaumburg, IL: La Leche League International, 1997.

4. Newman, Jack, MD, and Teresa Pitman. *The Ultimate Breastfeeding Book of Answers: The Most Comprehensive Problem-Solution Guide to*

Breastfeeding from the Foremost Expert in North America. Rocklin, CA: Prima Publishing, 2000.

5. WHO and UNICEF joint statement. *Protecting, Promoting and Supporting Breast-feeding: The Special Role of Maternity Services.* Geneva, Switzerland: WHO; 1989.

6. AAP policy statement. "Breastfeeding and the use of human milk." *Pediatrics,* vol. 100, no. 6 (December 1997): 1035–1039.

7. Griggs, Barbara. *Green Pharmacy: A History of Herbal Medicine.* London: Robert Hale, 1981.

8. La Leche League International. *The Womanly Art of Breastfeeding.*

9. Newman and Pitman. *The Ultimate Breastfeeding Book of Answers.*

10. Ibid.

11. La Leche League International. *The Womanly Art of Breastfeeding.*

$\mathscr{A}$ppendix A

Breastfeeding and Related Topics

Bengston, Diane. *How Weaning Happens.* Schaumburg, IL: La Leche League International, 2000.

Bumgarner, Norma Jane. *Mothering Your Nursing Toddler.* Rev. ed. Schaumburg, IL: La Leche League International, 1982.

Genna, Catherine Watson, ed. *Supporting Sucking Skills in Breastfeeding Infants.* Sudbury, MA: Jones and Bartlett, 2008.

Gotsch, Gwen. *Breastfeeding Your Premature Baby.* Schaumburg, IL: La Leche League International, 1999.

Gotsch, Gwen, and William Sears. *Breastfeeding Pure and Simple.* Rev. ed. Schaumburg, IL: La Leche League International, 1994.

Gotsch, Gwen, Anwar Fazal, and Judy Torgus, eds. *The Womanly Art of Breastfeeding.* 6th ed. Schaumburg, IL: La Leche League International, 1997.

Granju, Katie Allison, with Betsy Kennedy. *Attachment Parenting: Instinctive Care for Your Baby and Young Child.* New York: Pocket Books, 1999.

Humphrey, Sheila. "Sage Advice about Herbs." *Leaven.* Vol. 34, no. 3 (June–July 1998): 43–47.

Humphrey, Sheila I., and Dennis J. McKenna. "Herbs and Breastfeeding." *Breastfeeding Abstracts.* Vol. 17, no. 2 (November 1997): 11–12.

Jacobsen, Hilary. *Mother Food: A Breastfeeding Mother's Guide with Lactogenic Foods and Herbs: Build Milk Supply, Boost Immunity, Lift Depression, Detox, Lose Weight, Optimize a Baby's IQ, and Reduce Colic and Allergies.* Otsego, MI: Pagefree Press, 2004.

Johnson, Roberta, ed. *Whole Foods for the Whole Family Cookbook.* 2nd ed. Schaumburg, IL: La Leche League International, 1993.

Kerkoff Gromada, Karen. *Mothering Multiples: Breastfeeding and Caring for Twins or More!* 2nd ed. Schaumburg, IL: La Leche League International, 1999.

Kippley, Sheila. *Breastfeeding and Natural Child Spacing: How Ecological Breastfeeding Spaces Babies.* Rev. ed. Cincinnati: Couple to Couple League, 1999.

Mohrbacher, Nancy, and Katherine Kendall-Tackett. *Breastfeeding Made Simple.* Oakland, CA: New Harbinger, 2005.

Newman, Jack, MD, and Teresa Pitman. *The Ultimate Breastfeeding Book of Answers: The Most Comprehensive Problem-Solution Guide to Breastfeeding from the Foremost Expert in North America.* Rocklin, CA: Prima Publishing, 2000.

Peterson, Debra Stewart. *Breastfeeding the Adopted Baby.* Rev. ed. San Antonio: Corona Publishing, 1995.

Pryor, Gayle. *Nursing Mother, Working Mother: The Essential Guide for Breastfeeding and Staying Close to Your Baby after You Return to Work.* Boston: Harvard Common Press, 1997.

Sears, Martha, and William Sears. *The Breastfeeding Book: Everything You Need to Know about Nursing Your Child from Birth through Weaning.* Boston: Little, Brown, 2000.

Trevathan, Wendy R., E. O. Smith, and James J. McKenna, eds. *Evolutionary Medicine.* Oxford, NY: Oxford University Press, 1999.

West, Diana. *Defining Your Own Success: Breastfeeding after Breast Reduction Surgery.* Schaumburg, IL: La Leche League International, 2001.

West, Diana, and Lisa Marasco. *The Breastfeeding Mother's Guide to Making More Milk.* New York, NY: McGraw-Hill, 2009.

Winstein, Merryl. *Your Fertility Signals: Using Them to Achieve or Avoid Pregnancy.* St. Louis: Smooth Stone Press, 1994.

Women and Children's Herbal Books

Castro, Miranda. *Homeopathy for Pregnancy, Birth and Your Baby's First Year.* New York: St. Martin's Press, 1993.

Gladstar, Rosemary. *Herbal Healing for Women: Simple Home Remedies for Women of All Ages.* New York: Simon and Schuster, 1993.

Gladstar, Rosemary. *Herbal Remedies for Children's Health.* Pownal, VT: Storey Books, 1999.

Kemper, Kathi J., MD. *The Holistic Pediatrician: A Parent's Comprehensive Guide to Safe and Effective Therapies for the 25 Most Common Childhood Ailments.* New York: HarperPerennial, 1996.

Romm, Aviva Jill. *Naturally Healthy Babies and Children: A Commonsense Guide to Herbal Remedies, Nutrition, and Health.* Pownal, VT: Storey Books, 2000.

Romm, Aviva Jill. *The Natural Pregnancy Book: Herbs, Nutrition, and Other Holistic Choices.* Freedom, CA: Crossing Press, 1997.

Scott, Julian, and Susan Scott. *Natural Medicine for Women.* New York: Avon Books, 1991.

Soule, Deb. *A Woman's Book of Herbs.* New York: Citadel Press, 1995.

Tisserand, Maggie. *Aromatherapy for Women: A Practical Guide to Essential Oils for Health and Beauty.* Rochester, VT: Healing Arts Press, 1988.

Weed, Susun S. *Healing Wise.* Woodstock, NY: Ash Tree Publishing, 1989.

Weed, Susun S. *Menopausal Years, the Wise Woman Way: Alternative Approaches for Women 30–90.* Wise Woman Herbal Series, Book 5. Woodstock, NY: Ash Tree Publishing, 1992.

Weed, Susun S. *Wise Woman Herbal for the Childbearing Year.* Woodstock, NY: Ash Tree Publishing, 1986.

White, Linda B., MD, and Sunny Mavor. *Kids, Herbs, Health: A Parent's Guide to Natural Remedies.* Loveland, CO: Interweave Press, 1999.

General Herbal and Alternative Therapies

Culpeper, Nicholas. *Culpeper's Herbal.* Facsimile ed. Hertfordshire, England: Wordsworth Editions, 1995.

Dossey, Larry, MD. *Reinventing Medicine: Beyond Mind-Body to a New Era of Healing.* New York: HarperCollins, 1999.

Duke, James A. *Dr. Duke's Essential Herbs.* Emmaus, PA: Rodale Press, 1999.

Duke, James A. *The Green Pharmacy.* Emmaus, PA: Rodale Press, 1997.

Grieve, Mrs. M. *A Modern Herbal, Vol I & II.* Facsimile ed. New York: Dover Publications, 1971.

Griggs, Barbara. *Green Pharmacy: A History of Herbal Medicine.* London: Robert Hale, 1981.

Hoffmann, David. *The New Holistic Herbal: A Herbal Celebrating the Wholeness of Life.* Dorset, England: Element Books, 1990.

Lawless, Julia. *The Illustrated Encyclopedia of Essential Oils.* Dorset, England: Element Books, 1995.

Mondoa, Emil I., MD, and Mindy Kitei. *Sugars That Heal: The New Healing Science of Glyconutrients.* New York: Ballantine, 2001.

Ody, Penelope. *The Complete Medicinal Herbal.* London: Dorling Kindersley, 1993.

Murray, Michael T. *The Healing Power of Herbs: The Enlightened Person's Guide to the Wonders of Medicinal Plants.* 2nd ed. Rocklin, CA: Prima Publishing, 1995.

Murray, Michael T. *Natural Alternatives to Over-the-Counter and Prescription Drugs.* New York: William Morrow, 1994.

Pelletier, Kenneth R. *The Best Alternative Medicine: What Works? What Doesn't?* New York: Simon and Schuster, 2000.

Riddle, John M. *Eve's Herbs: A History of Contraception and Abortion in the West.* Cambridge, MA: Harvard University Press, 1997.

Robbers, James E., and Varro E. Tyler. *Tyler's Herbs of Choice: The Therapeutic Use of Phytomedicinals.* New York: Haworth Herbal Press, 1999.

Roberts, Arthur J., MD, Mary E. O'Brien, MD, and Genell Subak-Sharpe, eds. *Nutraceuticals: The Complete Encyclopedia of Supplements, Herbs, Vitamins, and Healing Foods.* New York: Perigee Press, 2001.

Tyler, Varro E. *Herbs of Choice: The Therapeutic Use of Phytomedicinals.* Binghamton, NY: Pharmaceutical Products Press, 1994.

Tyler, Varro E. *The Honest Herbal: A Sensible Guide to the Use of Herbs and Related Remedies.* Binghamton, New York: Pharmaceutical Products Press, 1993.

Weil, Andrew, MD. *Health and Healing.* Boston: Houghton Mifflin, 1988.

Weil, Andrew, MD. *Spontaneous Healing: How to Discover and Enhance Your Body's Natural Ability to Maintain and Heal Itself.* New York: Alfred A. Knopf, 1995.

Wood, Matthew. *Vitalism: The History of Herbalism, Homeopathy, and Flower Essences.* Berkeley, CA: North Atlantic Books, 2000.

Zand, Janet, Allan Spreen, and James B. LaValle. *Smart Medicine for Healthier Living: A Practical A-to-Z Reference to Natural and Conventional Treatments for Adults.* Garden City Park, NY: Avery Publishing, 1999.

Standard Professional Reference Texts and Selected Articles

Bingel, Audrey S., and Norman R. Farnsworth. "Higher Plants as Potential Sources of Galactogogues." *Economic and Medicinal Plant Research*, vol. 6, ed. by H. Wagner, H. Hikino, and N. R. Farnsworth. New York: Academic Press, 1991.

Bisset, Norman Grainger, and Max Wichtl, eds. *Herbal Drugs and Phytopharmaceuticals: A Handbook for Practice on a Scientific Basis.* English ed. Boca Raton, FL: CRC Press, 2001

Blumenthal, M., et al., eds. *The Complete German Commission E Monographs: Therapeutic Guide to Herbal Medicine.* Translated by S. Klein and R. S. Rister. Austin, TX: American Botanical Council, 1998.

Brinker, Francis. *Herb Contraindications and Drug Interactions.* 2nd ed. Sandy, OR: Eclectic Medical Publications, 1998.

Duke, James A. *Handbook of Medicinal Herbs.* Boca Raton, FL: CRC Press, 1985.

Duke, James A. *Handbook of Medicinal Herbs.* 2nd ed. Boca Raton, FL: CRC Press, 2002.

Farnsworth, Norman R. "Relative Safety of Herbal Medicines." *Herbalgram* 29 (1993): 36A–H. (This article can be ordered through the American Botanical Council.)

Hale, Thomas. *Medications and Mother's Milk: A Manual of Lactation Pharmacology.* 10th ed. Amarillo, TX: Pharmasoft Medical Publishing, 2002.

Lawrence, Ruth, MD, and Robert Lawrence, MD. *Breastfeeding: A Guide to the Medical Profession.* 5th ed. St. Louis: Mosby Press, 1999.

Leung, Albert Y., and Steven Foster. *Encyclopedia of Common Natural Ingredients Used in Foods, Drugs, and Cosmetics.* 2nd ed. New York: John Wiley and Sons, 1996.

Libster, Martha. *Delmar's Integrative Herb Guide for Nurses.* Albany, NY: Delmar Press, 2002.

Lust, K. D., J. E. Brown, and W. Thomas. "Maternal Intake of Cruciferous Vegetables and Other Foods and Colic Symptoms in Exclusively Breast-fed Infants." *J. Amer. Dietetic Assoc.* Vol. 96, no. 1 (1996): 46–48.

McGuffin, Michael, Christopher Hobbs, Roy Upton, and Alicia Goldberg, eds. *American Herbal Products Association's Botanical Safety Handbook*. Boca Raton, FL: CRC Press, 1997.

McKenna, Dennis, Kenneth Jones, and Kerry Hughes, with Sheila Humphrey. *Botanical Medicines: The Desk Reference for Major Herbal Supplements*. 2nd ed. Binghamton, NY: Haworth Press, 2002.

Mills, Simon, and Kerry Bone. *Principles and Practice of Phytotherapy*. Edinburgh, Scotland: Churchill Livingstone, 1999.

Newall, C. A., L. A. Anderson, and J. D. Phillipson. *Herbal Medicines: A Guide for Health-Care Professionals*. London: Pharmaceutical Press, 1996.

Riordan, Jan, and Kathleen G. Auerbach, eds. *Breastfeeding and Human Lactation*. 2nd ed. Boston: Jones and Bartlett, 1999.

Schilcher, H. *Phytotherapy in Paediatrics: Handbook for Physicians and Pharmacists*. Stuttgart, Germany: Medpharm Scientific Publishers, 1997.

Swafford, S., and B. Berns. "Effect of Fenugreek on Breast Milk Volume." Annual Meeting Abstracts. *Academy of Breastfeeding Medicine News and Views*. Vol. 6, no. 3 (September 11–13, 2000).

Wren, R. C. *Potter's New Cyclopaedia of Botanical Drugs and Preparations*. Rev. by Elizabeth M. Williamson and Fred J. Evans. Essex, England: C. W. Daniel Publishers, 1988.

$\mathscr{A}$ppendix B

Breastfeeding

General Information and Support

Ask Lenore
Web site: www.asklenore.info
*Information and support for nursing an
adopted child.*

Association of Breastfeeding Mothers
P.O. Box 207, Bridgwater
Somerset TA6 7YT, United Kingdom
E-mail: abm@clara.net
Web site: home.clara.net/abm

Australian Breastfeeding Association
(formerly Nursing Mothers' Association
of Australia), P.O. Box 4000, Glen Iris,
Victoria 3146, Australia
Phone: +61 (03) 9885 0855

E-mail: info@breastfeeding.asn.au
Web site: www.breastfeeding.asn.au

Breastfeeding after Reduction
Web site: www.bfar.org
*A discussion group for women who have
had breast reduction surgery and are now,
or soon will be, breastfeeding.*

Dr. Jay Gordon
Web site: www.drjaygordon.com
*A well-known pediatrician and lactation
specialist, Dr. Jay Gordon offers natural
remedies for thrush and other conditions.*

Handouts by Jack Newman, MD
Web site: www.breastfeedingonline.com/
newman.shtml
*Dr. Jack Newman is a pediatrician and an
internationally recognized expert in
lactation. He freely shares articles,*

treatment protocols, and the patient handouts he has developed through his years of practice with breastfeeding mothers.

Kathleen Kendall-Tackett, PhD
Web site: www.granitescientific.com
Kathleen Kendall-Tackett, PhD, is a lactation specialist and psychologist who specializes in helping mothers with post-partum depression. Her web pages offer information on a variety of topics, including depression, breastfeeding, child abuse and neglect, and disability.

La Leche League International
1400 N. Meacham Road, P.O.
Box 4079, Schaumburg, IL 60173-4808
Phone: 800-LALECHE [525-3243];
847-519-7730
Fax: 847-519-0035
Web site: www.lalecheleague.org
A nonprofit, nonsectarian volunteer organization dedicated to helping mothers who want to breastfeed their children. You can locate a La Leche League Group and Leader in your phone book, or call the 800 number above. The web site lists many (but not all) local groups, offers extensive information on all aspects of breastfeeding, and allows you to connect with a Leader through e-mail. A complete catalog of reliable books, information sheets, and other resources is available through your local La Leche League, by mail, or online.

La Leche League of Canada
18C Industrial Drive, P.O. Box 29,
Chesterville, Ontario K0C 1H0, Canada
Phone: 800-665-4324; 613-448-1842
Fax: 613-448-1845
E-mail: laleche@igs.net
Web site: www.lalecheleaguecanada.ca

National Childbirth Trust
Alexandra House, Oldham Terrace,
Acton, London W3 6NH, UK
Phone: +44 (0870) 770 3236;
+44 (0870) 444 8708
Fax: +44 (0870) 770 3237
Web site: www.nctpregnancyandbabycare.
   com/nct-online/
Free breastfeeding counselors throughout the United Kingdom.

Breastfeeding Professionals

Academy of Breastfeeding Medicine
191 Clarksville Road, Princeton
Junction, NJ 08550
Phone: 877-836-9947, ext. 25;
609-799-6327
Fax: 609-799-7032
E-mail: ABM@bfmed.org
Web site: www.bfmed.org

American Academy of Pediatrics
141 Northwest Point Boulevard, Elk
Grove Village, IL 60007
Phone: 800-433-9016
Web site: www.aap.org/policy/0063.html
For the AAP policy statement "Transfer of drugs and other chemicals into human milk," Pediatrics, *vol. 108, no. 3 (9/01): 776–789, go to* www.aap.org/policy/0063.html. *For the AAP policy statement "Breastfeeding and the use of human milk,"* Pediatrics, *vol. 100, no. 6 (12/97): 1035–1039, go to* www.aap.org/policy/re9729.html.

The Breastfeeding and Human Lactation Study Center
University of Rochester School of
Medicine and Dentistry, Dept. of
Pediatrics, Box 777, Rochester, NY 14642
Phone: 716-275-0088

Fax: 716-461-3614
Web site: www.cdc.gov/breastfeeding/
    compend-bhlsc.htm

Bright Future Lactation Resource Center
6540 Cedarview Court, Dayton,
OH 45459
Phone: 800-667-8939; 937-438-9458
Fax: 937-438-3229
E-mail: lindaJ@bflrc.com
Web site: www.bflrc.com

Dr. Jack Newman's Breastfeeding Clinics
Breastfeeding Program, Hospital for
Sick Children, 555 University Avenue,
Toronto, Ontario M5G 1X8, Canada
Phone: 416-813-5757
Web site: www.sickkids.on.ca

**Human Milk Banking Association of
North America**
1500 Sunday Drive, Suite 102,
Raleigh, NC 27607
Phone: 888-232-8809; 508-888-4041
Fax: 508-888-8050
Web site: www.hmbana.com
*Provides contact information for milk bank
locations in the United States and Canada.
There are currently six banks in the United
States and one in Canada. For information
on how to donate or acquire breast milk,
contact a lactation consultant as well as the
nearest milk bank.*

**International Lactation Consultant
Association**
1500 Sunday Drive, Suite 102, Raleigh,
NC 27607
Phone: 919-861-5577
Fax: 919-787-4916
E-mail: info@ilca.org
Web site: www.ILCA.org

World Health Organization (WHO)
Avenue Appia 20, 1211 Geneva 27,
Switzerland
Phone: +41 (022) 791 2111
Fax: +41 (022) 791 3111
E-mail: info@who.int
Web site: www.who.int/en/

Pumps, Devices, and Other Breastfeeding Aids

Ameda Breastfeeding Products
c/o Hollister Incorporated, 2000
Hollister Drive, Libertyville, IL 60048
Phone: 877-992-6332
E-mail: us.ameda.feedback@ameda.com
Web site: www.ameda.com/index.asp

Lact-Aid International, Inc.
P.O. Box 1066, Athens, TN 37371-1066
Phone 866-866-1239; 423-744-9090
Fax: 423-744-9116
Website: www.lact-aid.com
Email: orders@lact-aid.com
*The Lact-Aid Nursing Trainer System
supplements at the breast.*

La Leche League International
1400 N. Meacham Road, P.O. Box 4079
Schaumburg, IL 60173-4808
Phone: 800-LALECHE [525-3243];
847-519-7730
Fax: 847-519-0035
Web site: www.lalecheleague.org
*The La Leche League catalog contains a
wide selection of breastfeeding aids,
including breast shells, nipple everters, feeding cups, Lact-Aid and Medela supplement
tube feeders, finger-feeder devices, purified
lanolin, milk storage accessories, nursing
pads, baby slings, and nursing pillows.*

Medela, Inc.
1101 Corporate Drive, P.O. Box 660,
McHenry, IL 60050
Phone: 800-435-8316
Web site: www.medela.com
Offers breast pumps and breastfeeding accessories.

Whisper Wear
2221 Newmarket Parkway, Suite 136,
Marietta, GA 30067
Phone: 770-984-0905
Fax: 770-984-0587
Web site: www.whisperwear.com

Whittlestone
P.O. Box 2237, Antioch, CA 94531
Phone: 877-608-MILK [6455]
Fax: 877-609-MILK [6455]
Web site: www.whittlestone.com

Herb Companies with Lactation Products

Birth and Breastfeeding Resources
E-mail: mrturner@peedeeworld.net
Web site: www.birthandbreastfeeding.com
Mechell Turner is a traditionally trained herbalist and IBCLC lactation consultant. She offers information, lactation services, and a wide variety of prenatal, birth, postpartum, and herbal breastfeeding products. Galactogogue products include simple tinctures (alfalfa, anise, black cohosh, blessed thistle, borage, caraway, chasteberry, dandelion, dill, fennel, fenugreek, goat's rue, hops, marshmallow root, milk thistle leaf, motherwort, nettle, raspberry leaf, schisandra, wild lettuce) and combination tinctures, including Ancient One's Formula (anise, dill, fennel, fenugreek), LC's Proprietary

Blend (blessed thistle, fenugreek), Milk-In Formula (blessed thistle, borage, fenugreek, goat's rue, raspberry leaf), Mega-Milk Formula (blessed thistle, borage, red raspberry), Let-down Formula (black cohosh, motherwort, schisandra), and Let-down Formula F (black cohosh, fenugreek, motherwort, schisandra). Antigalactogogue products include sage tincture and Dry-Up-Quick (sage and parsley combined with the homeopathic remedy Lac caninum 30c). Turner also sells Anti-Puffy Formula for postpartum edema (corn silk, dandelion) and Mastitis/Yeast Formula (echinacea, goldenseal, myrrh, and colloidal silver combined with these homeopathic remedies: phytolacca 30c, belladonna 200c, echinacea 6x, sulfur 6x).

Motherlove Herbal Company
P.O. Box 101, Laporte, CO 80535
Phone: 888-209-8321; 970-493-2892
E-mail: mother@motherlove.com
Web site: www.motherlove.com
A diverse set of herbal products for pregnancy, birth, breastfeeding, postpartum healing, and baby care. Galactogogue products include More Milk (blessed thistle, nettle, fennel), More Milk Plus (fenugreek, blessed thistle, nettle, fennel) Fenugreek Tincture, and Goat's Rue Tincture. Galactogogue products for pregnant women include More Milk Two (raspberry leaf, nettle, alfalfa) and Tea for Two (alfalfa, nettle, raspberry leaf, spearmint, lemon balm). Motherlove also offers Sage Tincture, an antigalactogogue, as well as Breast Compress, ready-made packets for engorgement, plugged ducts, and other breast discomforts (mullein, marshmallow, chamomile, elder, yarrow).

Traditional Medicinals
4515 Ross Road, Sebastopol, CA 95472
Phone: 800-543-4372
Web site: www.traditionalmedicinals.com
*This company posts safety and quality control
information on its web site, providing a good
example of what goes into a high-quality
product. Traditional Medicinals sells a
number of products designed for reproductive
health, including a galactogogue tea called
Mother's Milk Tea (fennel, anise, coriander,
spearmint, lemongrass, lemon verbena,
marshmallow, blessed thistle, fenugreek),
which is widely available in stores.*

Turtle Island Herbs
c/o Lotus Light, P.O. Box 1008, Silver
Lake, WI 53170
Phone: 800-548-3824; 262-889-8501
Fax: 800-905-6887; 262-889-8591
E-mail: turtleisland@lotuslight.com
Web site: www.lotuslight.com
*Makers of a galactogogue tincture called
Nursing Mother's Support (fennel, blessed
thistle, raspberry, burdock, red clover).*

Weleda, Inc.
USA Division, 175 North Route 9W,
Congers, NY 10920
Phone: 800-241-1030
E-mail: info@weleda.com
Web sites: usa.weleda.com;
             www.weleda.com
*Sells high-quality herbal and homeopathic
products all over the world. Weleda's
galactogogue tea, called Nursing Tea
(caraway, fennel, anise, nettle), can be
ordered through its USA web site. This tea
has been sold for decades in Germany.*

Breastfeeding Advocates

Baby Milk Action
23 St. Andrews Street, Cambridge
CB2 3AX, United Kingdom
Phone: +44 (01223) 464 420
Fax: +44 (01223) 464 417
Web site: www.babymilkaction.org

Geneva Infant Feeding Association
C.P. 157, 1211 Geneva 19, Switzerland
Phone: +41 (022) 798 9164
Fax: +41 (022) 798 4443
E-mail: info@gifa.org
Web site: www.gifa.org

INFACT Canada
6 Trinity Square, Toronto,
Ontario M5G 1B1, Canada
Phone: 416-595-9819
Fax: 416-591-9355
E-mail: info@infactcanada.ca
Web site: www.infactcanada.ca

**International Baby Food Action
Network (IBFAN)**
INFACT Canada, P.O. Box 781,
10 Trinity Square, Toronto, Ontario
M5G 1B1, Canada
Phone: 416-595-9819
Fax: 416-591-9355
E-mail: infact@ftn.net
Web site: www.ibfan.org
*A network of more than 150 citizen groups
in over ninety countries. You can contact
the World Alliance for Breastfeeding Action
through the above web site.*

**World Alliance for Breastfeeding
Action (WABA)**
P.O. Box 1200, 10850 Penang, Malaysia
Phone: +60 (04) 658 4816

Fax: +60 (04) 657 2655

E-mail: secr@waba.po.my

Web site: www.waba.org.br/index.html

Parenting Resources

Attached Mamas

P.O. Box 55058, Virginia Beach,
VA 23471-0058

Phone: 877-839-9847

Fax: 877-839-9847

Web site: www.attachedmamas.com

Offers a variety of natural products for pregnancy, breastfeeding, and parenting, including breastfeeding products from a number of herb companies.

Breastfeeding.com

Web site: www.breastfeeding.com

Offers links to parenting and breastfeeding resources.

The Breastfeeding Stories Page

Web site: www.angelfire.com/nc2/bfstories

Stories and tips from nursing mothers.

The Compleat Mother Magazine: The Magazine of Pregnancy, Birth and Breastfeeding

Subscriptions, P.O. Box 209, Minot,
ND 58702

Phone: 710-852-2822

E-mail: jody@minot.com

Web site: www.compleatmother.com

Birth, breastfeeding, and parenting discussions offer the "uncut" version of reality.

Cuddle Karrier

1928 Wildflower Drive, Pickering,
Ontario L1V 7A7, Canada

Phone: 877-283-3535

Web site: www.cuddlekarrier.com

Sells an adjustable baby carrier, educational toys, and more.

Diana Designs

160 River Forest Drive, Sept. WP,
Fayetteville, GA 30214

E-mail: diana@dianadesigns.com

Web site: www.dianadesigns.com

Breastfeeding clothes and other items.

Doubletalk Newsletter

P.O. Box 412, Amelia, OH 45102

Phone: 513-231-TWIN [8946]

A newsletter for parents of multiples.

Kelly's Attachment Parenting

Web site: www.kellymom.com

Information about breastfeeding, attachment parenting, and the use of herbs and drugs during breastfeeding. Offers links to articles about fenugreek and other herbs of interest to breastfeeding mothers and their supporters. Especially recommended for those who want to know more about fenugreek.

Mothering Magazine

P.O. Box 1690, Santa Fe, NM 87504

Phone: 800-984-8116

Web site: www.mothering.com

Discusses health, personal, environmental, medical, and lifestyle issues.

National Association of At-Home Mothers

406 E. Buchanan Avenue, Fairfield,
IA 52556

Web site: www.AtHomeMothers.com

Support for at-home mothers. Offers articles, an online newsletter, and the only magazine published exclusively for mothers at home.

StorkNet
Web site: www.storknet.com
Well-organized web site offers links to
articles, books, and other resources on
pregnancy, doulas, breastfeeding, attachment
parenting, multiples parenting, working
and parenting, single parenting, and more.

Fertility, Pregnancy, and Birth

American Academy of Family Physicians
P.O. Box 11210, Shawnee Mission,
KS 66207-1210
Phone: 800-274-2237; 913-906-6000
Web site: www.aafp.org

American Academy of Husband-Coached Childbirth
P.O. Box 5224, Sherman Oaks,
CA 91413-5224
Phone: 800-4-A-BIRTH [422-4784]
Web site: www.bradleybirth.com
Information on the Bradley Method of
childbirth.

American Academy of Pediatrics
141 Northwest Point Boulevard
Elk Grove Village, IL 60007
Phone: 800-433-9016
Web site: www.aap.org

American College of Nurse-Midwives
818 Connecticut Avenue, N.W.,
Suite 900, Washington, DC 20006
Phone: 202-728-9860
Fax: 202-728-9897
Web site: www.acnm.org

The American College of Obstetricians and Gynecologists
409 12th Street, S.W., P.O. Box 96920,
Washington, DC 20090-6920
Web site: www.acog.com

Association of Women's Health, Obstetric and Neonatal Nurses
2000 L Street, N.W., Suite 740,
Washington, DC 20036
Phone: 800-673-8499 (United States);
800-245-0231 (Canada)
Fax: 202-728-0575
Web site: www.awhonn.org

Couple to Couple League
P.O. Box 111184, Cincinnati,
OH 45211-1184
Phone: 513-471-2000
Fax: 513-557-2449
Web site: www.ccli.org
This organization is dedicated to
educating couples about natural methods
of birth control.

Doulas of North America
P.O. Box 626, Jasper, IN 47547
Phone: 888-788-DONA [3662]
Fax: 812-634-1491
Web site: www.dona.org

Institute for Reproductive Health
Georgetown University,
4301 Connecticut Avenue, N.W.,
Suite 310, Washington, DC 20008
Phone: 202-687-1392
Fax: 202-537-7450
E-mail: irhinfo@georgetown.edu
Web site: www.irh.org

International Childbirth Education Association Bookcenter
P.O. Box 20048, Minneapolis, MN 55420
Phone: 800-624-4934; 612-854-8660
Fax: 612-854-8772
Web site: www.icea.org/book.htm

International Confederation of Midwives
Eisenhowerlaan 138, 2517 KN
The Hague, The Netherlands
Phone: +31 (070) 306 0520
Fax: +31 (070) 355 5651
Web site: www.internationalmidwives.org

Midwifery Education and Accreditation Council
222 West Birch, Flagstaff, AZ 86001
Phone: 928-214-0997
E-mail: meac@altavista.net
Web site: www.meacschools.org

Midwives Alliance of North America
4805 Lawrenceville Highway,
Suite 116–279, Lilburn, GA 30047
Phone: 888-923-MANA [6262]
E-mail: Info@mana.org
Web site: www.mana.org

Midwives Information and Resource Service
9 Elmdale Road, Clifton,
Bristol BS8 1SL, United Kingdom
Phone: +44 (0117) 925 1791
Fax: +44 (0117) 925 1792
Web site: www.midirs.org

North American Registry of Midwives
5257 Rosestone Drive, Lilburn,
GA 30047
Phone: 888-84-BIRTH [842-4784]
E-mail: info@narm.org
Web site: www.narm.org

Perinatal Education Association
98 E. Franklin Street, Suite B,
Centerville, OH 45459
Phone: 866-88-BIRTH [882-4784];
937-312-0544
Fax: 937-312-0545
E-mail: info@birthsource.com
Web site: www.birthsource.com
Information about pregnancy and childbirth.

Royal College of Midwives
15 Mansfield Street, London
W1M OBE, United Kingdom
Phone: +44 (020) 7312 3535
Fax: +44 (020) 7312 3536
Web site: www.rcm.org.uk

Herbs and Nutrition

Herbal Information and Education

The American Botanical Council
P.O. Box 144345, Austin,
TX 78714-4345
Phone: 512-926-4900
Fax: 512-926-2345
E-mail: abc@herbalgram.org
Web site: www.herbalgram.org
A nonprofit organization dedicated to educating the public about herbs.

American Herbalists Guild
1931 Gaddis Road, Canton, GA 30115
Phone: 770-751-6021
Fax: 770-751-7472
E-mail: ahgoffice@earthlink.net
Web site: americanherbalistsguild.com
Visit the web site for a list of practitioners who meet AHG's criteria for training and clinical experience.

American Herb Association
Quarterly Newsletter
P.O. Box 1673, Nevada City, CA 95959
Phone: 530-265-9552
Web site: www.ahaherb.com

Canadian Herbal Practitioners Newsletter
302–1220 Kensington Road NW,
Calgary, Alberta T2N 3P5, Canada

Complementary Health Studies
Programme
Dept. of Lifelong Learning, School of
Education, University of Exeter,
St. Luke's Campus, Heavitree Road,
Exeter EX1 2LU, United Kingdom
Phone: +44 (01392) 262 898
Fax: +44 (01392) 433 828
E-mail: CHS@exeter.ac.uk
Web site: www.exeter.ac.uk/chs

Dr. Duke's Phytochemical and
Ethnobotanical Databases
Web site: www.ars-grin.gov/duke/
This free-access database of plant chemicals
and their known activities represents
decades of research and compilation by well-
known USDA *botanist (retired) James A.*
Duke. Includes both folk and medicinal uses
for plants. Provides reference sources for all
information in the database, as well as links
to other herbal and nutritional databases.

HerbalGram
American Botanical Council,
P.O. Box 144345, Austin,
TX 78714-4345
Phone: 512-926-4900
Fax: 512-926-2345
E-mail: abc@herbalgram.org
Web site: www.herbalgram.org

Herbal Green Pages
P.O. Box 245, Silver Spring, MD 17575
Phone: 717-393-3295
E-mail: herbworld@aol.com
Web site: www.herbworld.com/index.htm

Journal of the American Herbalists Guild
American Herbalists Guild,
1931 Gaddis Road, Canton, GA 30115
Phone: 770-751-6021
Fax: 770-751-7472
Web site: americanherbalistsguild.com

Kelly's Attachment Parenting
Web site: www.kellymom.com
Offers links to articles about fenugreek and
other herbs of interest to breastfeeding
mothers and their supporters. Especially
recommended for those who want to know
more about fenugreek.

A Mini-Course in Medical Botany
James A. Duke, Ethnobotanist
The Herbal Village, 8210 Murphy
Road, Fulton, MD 20759
Web site: www.ars-grin.gov/duke/syllabus/
Excellent reading available online.

National Institute of Medical Herbalists
56 Longbrook Street, Exeter,
Devon EX4 6AH, United Kingdom
Phone: +44 (01392) 426 022
Fax: +44 (01392) 498 963
E-mail: nimh@ukexeter.freeserve.co.uk
Web site: www.nimh.org.uk

Native American
Ethnobotanical Database
Web site: www.umd.umich.edu/
cgi-bin/herb
Database covering the foods, drugs, dyes,
and fibers of the native peoples of North

America. Provided by Dan Moerman, professor of anthropology at the University of Michigan–Dearborn.

United Plant Savers
P.O. Box 77, Guysville, OH 45735
Phone: 740-662-0041
Fax. 740-662.0242
E-mail: info@unitedplantsavers.org
Web site: www.unitedplantsavers.org

World Health Organization (WHO)
Dr. Xiaorui Zhang
Traditional Medicine
Essential Drugs and Medicines Policy
Avenue Appia 20, 1211 Geneva 27,
Switzerland
Fax: +41 (022) 791 4730
E-mail: trm@who.int
Web site: www.who.int/en/

Nutrition

DoctorYourself.Com
Andrew Saul, Number 8 Van Buren
Street, Holley, NY 14470
Phone: 585-638-5357
E-mail: drsaul@doctoryourself.com
Web site: www.doctoryourself.com/
    index.html
A "renegade" information source.

DrWeil.com
Andrew Weil, MD
Web site: www.drweil.com
Offers information on integrative medicine, including nutrition and other health topics. Dr. Weil is an educator and leading advocate for integrative medicine.

Food and Nutrition Information Center
Agricultural Research Service, USDA

National Agricultural Library,
Room 105, 10301 Baltimore Avenue,
Beltsville, MD 20705-2351
Phone: 301-504-5719
Fax: 301-504-6409
TTY: 301-504-6856
E-mail: fnic@nal.usda.gov
Web site: www.nal.usda.gov/fnic/
Collects and disseminates information about food and human nutrition.

Nutrient Data Laboratory
Agricultural Research Service, Beltsville
Human Nutrition Research Center,
10300 Baltimore Avenue, Building 005,
Room 107, BARC-West, Beltsville,
MD 20705-2350
Phone: 301-504-0630
Fax: 301-504-0632
E-mail: jholden@rbhnrc.usda.gov
Web site: www.nal.usda.gov/fnic/
    foodcomp
Maintains authoritative databases on nutrition and food composition.

Vegetarian Times Magazine
Subscriber Service Department,
P.O. Box 420235, Palm Coast,
FL 32142-0235
Phone: 877-717-8923
Web site: www.vegetariantimes.com
Publishes recipes as well as articles on alternative medicine and nutrition.

Complementary and Alternative Medicine

General Information and Support

American Holistic Health Association
P.O. Box 17400, Anaheim,

CA 92817-7400
Phone: 714-779-6152
E-mail: mail@ahha.org
Web site: www.healthy.net/ahha

American Self-Help Group Clearinghouse
100 Hanover Avenue, Suite 202,
Cedar Knolls, NJ 07927
Phone: 973-326-6789
Fax: 973-326-9467
Web site: www.selfhelpgroups.org
Puts people in touch with a variety of support groups throughout the United States.

DrWeil.com
Andrew Weil, MD
Web site: www.drweil.com
Offers information on integrative medicine, including nutrition and other health topics. Dr. Weil is an educator and leading advocate for integrative medicine.

Aromatherapy

Aromatherapy Institute of Research
P.O. Box 2345, Fair Oaks, CA 95628
Phone: 916-965-7546
Fax: 916-962-3272
Web site: www.leydet.com

International Federation of Aromatherapists
182 Chiswick High Road,
London W4 1PP, United Kingdom
Phone: +44 (020) 8742 2605
E-mail: office@ifaroma.org
Web site: www.ifaroma.org

The National Association for Holistic Aromatherapy
4509 Interlake Avenue North, No. 233,
Seattle, WA 98103-6773

Phone: 888-ASK-NAHA [275-6242];
206-547-2164
Fax: 206-547-2680
E-mail: info@naha.org
Web site: www.naha.org

Homeopathy and Flower Essences

American Institute of Homeopathy
801 North Fairfax Street, Suite 306,
Alexandria, VA 22314
Phone: 888-445-9988
Web site: www.homeopathyusa.org
While the American Institute of Homeopathy is a trade organization, nonprofessionals can access its member directory through its web site.

The Bach Centre
Mount Vernon, Bakers Lane, Sotwell,
Oxon OX10 0PZ, United Kingdom
Phone: +44 (01491) 834 678
Fax: +44 (01491) 825 022
E-mail: centre@bachcentre.com
Web site: www.bachcentre.com

Faculty of Homeopathy
British Homeopathic Association,
15 Clerkenwell Close, London
EC1R 0AA, United Kingdom
Phone: +44 (020) 7566 7800
Fax: +44 (020) 7566 7815
Web site: www.trusthomeopathy.org/
faculty/fac_over.html

Flower Essence Society
P.O. Box 459, Nevada City, CA 95959
Phone: 800-736-9222
Fax: 530-265-0584
E-mail: mail@flowersociety.org
Web site: www.flowersociety.org

National Center for Homeopathy
801 North Fairfax Street, Suite 306,
Alexandria, VA 22314
Phone: 877-624-0613; 703-548-7790
Fax: 703-548-7792
E-mail: info@homeopathic.org
Web site: www.homeopathic.org
Publishes Homeopathy Today; *describes
recognized homeopathy credentials; lists
practitioners and study groups.*

Society of Homeopaths
4a Artizan Road, Northhampton
NN1 4HU, United Kingdom
Phone: +44 (01604) 621 400
Fax: +44 (01604) 622 622
Web site: www.homeopathy-soh.org

Naturopathy

**The American Association of
Naturopathic Physicians**
3201 New Mexico Avenue, N.W.,
Suite 350, Washington, DC 20016
Phone: 866-538-2267; 202-895-1392
Fax: 202-274-1992
Web site: www.naturopathic.org

**Canadian College of
Naturopathic Medicine**
1255 Sheppard Avenue East, North
York, Ontario M2K 1E2, Canada
Phone: 416-498-1255
Fax: 416-498-1576
E-mail: info@ccnm.edu
Web site: www.ccnm.edu

Canadian Naturopathic Association
1255 Sheppard Avenue East, North
York, Ontario M2K 1E2, Canada

Phone: 800-551-4381; 416-496-8633
Fax: 416-496-8634
E-mail: info@naturopathicassoc.ca
Web site: www.naturopathicassoc.ca

**General Council and Register
of Naturopaths**
Goswell House, 2 Goswell Road,
Somerset BA16 0JG, United Kingdom
Phone: +44 (08707) 456 984
Fax: +44 (08707) 456 985
E-mail: admin@naturopathy.org.uk
Web site: www.naturopathy.org.uk

Eastern Medicine

**The Acupuncture and Oriental
Medicine Alliance**
6405 43rd Avenue Court N.W., Suite B,
Northwest Gig Harbor, WA 98335
Phone: 253-851-6896
Fax: 253-851-6883
Web site: www.aomalliance.org

**Acupuncture Foundation of
Canada Institute**
2131 Lawrence Avenue East, Suite 204,
Scarborough, Ontario M1R 5G4, Canada
Phone: 416-752-3988
Fax: 416-752-4398
E-mail: info@afcinstitute.com
Web site: www.afcinstitute.com

**American Association of Oriental
Medicine**
5530 Wisconsin Avenue, Suite 1210,
Chevy Chase, MD 20815
Phone: 888-500-7999; 301-941-1061
Fax: 301-986-9313
E-mail: info@aaom.org
Web site: www.aaom.org

The Ayurvedic Institute
P.O. Box 23445, Albuquerque,
NM 87192-1445
Phone: 505-291-9698
Fax: 505-294-7572
Web site: www.ayurveda.com

British Acupuncture Council
63 Jeddo Road, London W12 9HQ,
United Kingdom
Phone: +44 (020) 8735 0400
E-mail: info@acupuncture.org.uk
Web site: www.acupuncture.org.uk

**National Certification Commission for
Acupuncture and Oriental Medicine**
11 Canal Center Plaza, Suite 300,
Alexandria, VA 22314
Phone: 703-548-9004
Fax: 703-548-9079
E-mail: info@nccaom.org
Web site: www.nccaom.org

The Register of Chinese Herbal Medicine
Office 5, Ferndale Business Centre,
1 Exeter Street, Norwich NR2 4QB,
United Kingdom
Phone: +44 (01603) 623 994
Fax: +44 (01603) 667 557
E-mail: herbmed@rchm.co.uk
Web site: www.rchm.co.uk

Osteopathy and Chiropractic Care

American Academy of Osteopathy
3500 DePauw Boulevard, Suite 1080,
Indianapolis, IN 46268-1136
Phone: 317-879-1881
Fax: 317-879-0568
Web site: www.academyofosteopathy.org/

American Chiropractic Association
1701 Clarendon Boulevard, Arlington,
VA 22209
Phone: 800-986-4636; 703-276-8800
Fax: 703-243-2593
Web site: www.amerchiro.org

Canadian Chiropractic Association
1396 Eglinton Avenue West, Toronto,
Ontario M6C 2E4, Canada
Phone: 416-781-7344
E-mail: ccachiro@ccachiro.org
Web site: www.ccachiro.org

The Cranial Academy
8202 Clearvista Parkway, Suite 9D,
Indianapolis, IN 46255
Phone: 317-594-0411
Fax: 317-594-9299
Web site: www.cranialacademy.org

**The Craniosacral Therapy Association
of North America**
E-mail: info@craniosacraltherapy.org
Web site: www.craniosacraltherapy.org

General Osteopathic Council
Osteopathy House, 176 Tower Bridge
Road, London SE1 3LU, United Kingdom
Phone: +44 (020) 7357 6655
Fax: +44 (020) 7357 0011
Web site: www.osteopathy.org.uk

**International Chiropractic
Pediatric Association**
327 North Middletown Road, Media,
PA 19063
Phone: 610-565-2360
E-mail: info@icpa4kids.com
Web site: www.icpa4kids.com

International Chiropractors Association
1110 North Glebe Road, Suite 1000,
Arlington, VA 22201
Phone: 800-423-4690; 703-528-5000
Fax: 703-528-5023
E-mail: chiro@chiropractic.org
Web site: www.chiropractic.org

**The Sutherland Cranial Teaching
Foundation of Australia and New Zealand**
P.O. Box 355, Edgecliff, New South
Wales 2027, Australia
Phone: +61 (02) 9299 1311
Fax: +61 (02) 9299 3195

Upledger Institute
11211 Prosperity Farms Road, Suite D-
325, Palm Beach Gardens, FL 33410
Phone: 561-622-4706
Fax: 561-622-4771
E-mail: upledger@upledger.com
Web site: www.upledger.com

Bodywork and Yoga

Acupressure Institute
1533 Shattuck Avenue, Berkeley,
CA 94709
Phone: 800-442-2232; 510-845-1059
Fax: 510-845-1496
E-mail: info@acupressure.com
Web site: www.acupressure.com

American Massage Therapy Association
820 Davis Street, Suite 100, Evanston,
IL 60201-4444
Phone: 847-864-0123
Fax: 847-864-1178
Web site: www.amtamassage.org

**American Organization for Bodywork
Therapies of Asia**
1010 Haddonfield-Berlin Road,
Suite 408, Voorhees, NJ 08043-3514
Phone: 856-782-1616
Fax: 856-782-1653
E-mail: aobta@prodigy.net
Web site: www.aobta.org

American Physical Therapy Association
1111 North Fairfax Street, Alexandria,
VA 22314-1488
Phone: 800-999-APTA [2782];
703-684-APTA [2782]
Fax: 703-684-7343
Web site: www.apta.org

**Associated Bodywork and
Massage Professionals**
1271 Sugarbush Drive, Evergreen,
CO 80439-7347
Phone: 800-458-ABMP [2267];
303-674-8478
Fax: 800-667-8260; 303-674-0859
E-mail: expectmore@abmp.com
Web site: www.abmp.com

**Australian Association of
Massage Therapists**
P.O. Box 358, Prahran, Victoria 3181,
Australia
Phone: +61 (03) 9510 3930
Fax: +61 (03) 9521 3209
E-mail: amta@amta.asn.au
Web site: www.amta.asn.au

The Ayurvedic Institute
P.O. Box 23445, Albuquerque,
NM 87192-1445
Phone: 505-291-9698
Fax: 505-294-7572
Web site: www.ayurveda.com

The British Massage Therapy Council
17 Rymers Lane, Oxford,
Oxon OX4 3JU, United Kingdom
Phone: +44 (01865) 774 121
E-mail: info@bmtc.co.uk
Web site: www.bmtc.co.uk

The British Wheel of Yoga
25 Jermyn Street, Sleaford, Lincolnshire
NG34 7RU, United Kingdom
Phone: +44 (01529) 306 851
Fax: +44 (01529) 303 233
E-mail: office@bwy.org.uk
Web site: www.bwy.org.uk

**International Association of
Yoga Therapists**
2400A County Center Drive,
Santa Rosa, CA 95403
Phone: 707-566-9000
E-mail: mail@yrec.org
Web site: www.iayt.org

The Shiatsu Society
Eastland Court, St. Peters Road,
Rugby CV21 3QP, United Kingdom
Phone: +44 (0845) 130 4560
Fax: +44 (01788) 555 052
E-mail: admin@shiatsu.org
Web site: www.shiatsu.org

Guided Imagery and Relaxation Therapy

Academy for Guided Imagery
P.O. Box 2070, Mill Valley,
CA 94942
Phone: 800-726-2070; 415-389-9324
Fax: 415-389-9342
Web site: www. healthy.net/agi/
    index_explorer.html

British Autogenic Society
Royal London Homeopathic Hospital,
Greenwell Street, London W1W 5BP,
United Kingdom
Phone: +44 (020) 7383 5108
Fax: +44 (020) 7383 5108
Web site: www.autogenic-therapy.org.uk/
    index.htm

Dr. Kai Kermani
Holistic Health and Healing Center,
10 Connaught Hill, Loughton,
Essex IG10 4DU, United Kingdom
Phone: +44 (020) 8508 9712
Fax: +44 (020) 8508 9712
E-mail: healing@drkermani.freeserve.co.uk
Web site: www.healing-with-doctorkai
    .com

Institute of Noetic Sciences
101 San Antonio Road, Petaluma,
CA 94952
Phone: 707-775-3500
Fax: 707-781-7420
E-mail: membership@noetic.org
Web site: www.noetic.org

Mind Body Health Sciences
393 Dixon Road, Boulder, CO 80302
Phone: 303-440-8460

Hypnotherapy and Biofeedback

American Board of Hypnotherapy
2002 East McFadden Avenue,
Suite 100, Santa Ana, CA 92705
Phone: 800-872-9996
Fax: 714-245-9881
Web site: www.hypnosis.com

The American Society of Clinical Hypnosis
140 North Bloomingdale Road,
Bloomingdale, IL 60108-1017
Phone: 630-980-4740
Fax: 630-351-8490
E-mail: info@asch.net
Web site: www.asch.net

Association for Applied Psychophysiology and Biofeedback
10200 West 44th Avenue, Suite 304,
Wheat Ridge, CO 80033-2840
Phone: 800-477-8892; 303-422-8436
Fax: 303-422-8894
E-mail: aapb@resourcecenter.com
Web site: www.aapb.org

Biofeedback Certification Institute of America
10200 West 44th Avenue, Suite 310,
Wheat Ridge, CO 80033-2840
Phone: 303-420-2902
Fax: 303-422-8894
E-mail: bcia@resourcecenter.com
Web site: www.bcia.org

The National Council of Psychotherapists
P.O. Box 6072, Nottingham
NG9 BW, United Kingdom
Phone: +44 (0115) 913 1382
E-mail: ncphq@talk21.com
Web site: www.natcouncilof
          psychotherapists.org.uk

Society for Clinical and Experimental Hypnosis
P.O. Box 642114, Pullman,
WA 99164-2114
Phone: 509-335-7504
Fax: 509-335-2097

E-mail: sceh@wsu.edu
Web site: sunsite.utk.edu/IJCEH/
          scehframe.html

Tools for Wellness
9755 Independence Avenue,
Chatsworth, CA 91311-4318
Phone: 800-456-9887; 818-885-9090
Fax: 818-407-0850
Web site: www.toolsforwellness.com

Dance, Art, Music, Color, and Humor Therapies

American Art Therapy Association
1202 Allanson Road, Mundelein,
IL 60060-3808
Phone: 888-290-0878; 847-949-6064
Fax: 847-566-4580
E-mail: info@arttherapy.org
Web site: www.arttherapy.org

American Dance Therapy Association
2000 Century Plaza, Suite 108,
10632 Little Patuxent Parkway,
Columbia, MD 21044
Phone: 410-997-4040
Fax: 410-997-4048
E-mail: info@adta.org
Web site: www.adta.org

American Music Therapy Association
8455 Colesville Road, Suite 1000,
Silver Spring, MD 20910
Phone: 301-589-3300
Fax: 301-589-5175
E-mail: info@musictherapy.org
Web site: www.musictherapy.org

Association for Applied and Therapeutic Humor
1951 West Camelback Road,
Suite 445, Phoenix, AZ 85015
Phone: 602-995-1454
Fax: 602-995-1449
E-mail: office@aath.org
Web site: www.aath.org

British Society for Music Therapy
25 Rosslyn Avenue, East Barnet,
Herts EN4 8DH, United Kingdom
Phone: +44 (020) 8368 8879
Fax: +44 (020) 8368 8879
Web site: www.bsmt.org

California Institute of Integral Studies
1453 Mission Street, San Francisco,
CA 94103
Phone: 415-575-6100
E-mail: info@ciis.edu
Web site: www.ciis.edu

Certification Board for Music Therapists
506 East Lancaster Avenue,
Suite 102, Downingtown, PA 19335
Phone: 800-765-CBMT [2268]
E-mail: info@cbmt.org
Web site: www.cbmt.com

College of Chromotherapy
67 Farm Crescent, Wexham Court,
Slough, Berkshire SL2 5TQ,
United Kingdom
Phone: +44 (01753) 576 913

College of Syntonic Optometry
Web site: www.syntonicphototherapy
         .com

Dinshaw Health Society
100 Dinshaw Drive, Malaga,
NJ 08328
Phone: 609-692-4686

Hygeia Studios
Brook House, Avening, Tetbury,
Gloucestershire GL8 8NS,
United Kingdom
Phone: +44 (01453) 832 150
Fax: +44 (01453) 832 150

Omega Institute for Holistic Studies
150 Lake Drive, Rhinebeck,
NY 12572
Phone: 800-944-1001; 845-266-4444
Fax: 845-266-3769
Web site: www.eomega.org.

$\mathcal{A}$ppendix C

Before using any herb, you must familiarize yourself with dosage, preparation, effects, and safety concerns. The Plant Safety Table and the Galactogogue Herb Profiles are only a starting point; see chapters 3 and 4 for a full discussion of herb safety when breastfeeding.

Clearly, a breastfeeding mother needs to be cautious when using herbs or drugs. But what is meant by cautious? Just what specific actions should a mother take to be reasonably safe? Or to keep her baby safe? Keep in mind that the mother is the one most likely to suffer any adverse effects, not the baby. However, herbs with stronger effects or side effects are more likely to affect a young baby through breast milk than herbs that have mild effects.

Select your herbs carefully. Remember that some herbs, called galactogogues, have been used to increase milk production; others, called antigalactogogues, have been used to slow milk production or aid weaning. Many herbs are allergenic, which means they are known to cause allergic reactions, photosensitization, contact dermatitis, or other reactions. Also, a number of herbs are endangered in their natural habitat, so it's important to choose ethical herb companies that won't exploit endangered plants. All of these considerations are noted in the Plant Safety Table.

The table rates herbs according to their toxicity, interactions, contraindications, and other adverse effects (including overdose). It explains how different herbs can affect milk supply and which herbs are known allergens. Always remember that an herb could affect some breastfeeding dyads differently than expected, and that allergic reactions (in either the mother or infant) may occur with any substance, whether food, drug, or herb.

Safety Ratings

The letters A, B, C, D, or E indicate the degree of caution required for each herb. Letter A denotes relatively uncontroversial herbs, while E denotes herbs that are highly toxic:

A—No contraindications, side effects, drug interactions, or pregnancy-related safety issues have been identified. Generally considered safe when used appropriately.

B—May not be appropriate for self-use by some individuals or dyads, or may cause adverse effects if misused. Seek reliable safety and dose information.

C—Moderate potential for toxicity, mainly dose related. Seek an expert herbalist as well as a lactation consultation before using. Consider using safer herbs.

D—Use only with the supervision of a knowledgeable physician. Consult with a lactation specialist before use. These herbs are used to make prescription medications. The pharmaceutical forms may be safer in most instances, but not always. Do not use these herbs without the guidance of a supervising physician. Consider using safer herbs.

E—Avoid. Toxic plant with no justifiable medical use.

Most herbs (safety rating A) do not have the power to harm a breastfeeding infant unless misused by the mother. Stimulant herbs (mostly rated B) can make a baby fussy or sleepless. Other herbs (rated B or C) will offer benefits but have potentially serious effects if misused or used by certain individuals. Herbs rated B are generally considered safe to use if you are not pregnant, do not have a medical condition, and are not taking other medications. Herbs rated C require considerably more caution and skilled guidance for anyone to use safely. These herbs need to be put in context: How safe are they compared to other herbs? Are there safer alternatives? A few herbs (rated D) are used to make prescription medications that are considered safe for breastfeeding mothers (because they are always used with medical supervision). The herbs themselves are sometimes available over the counter, but their use is suggested only with medical supervision. A very few herbs (rated E) are inappropriate for any medicinal use: Those with toxins capable of causing irreversible harm to the body, or those that present serious risk even in proper doses.

The Plant Safety Table can give you only a rough measure of the relative safety for herbs. It does not tell you which herbs are okay to use when breastfeeding. This is something that simply cannot be determined by a book. Your health, your baby's health, and your breastfeeding situation will play a large role in determining which herbs are preferable for you. Be sure to let your doctor know about any herbs you are using, whether or not the physician is providing these treatments.

A Note on Pediatric Use
Oral use of herbs with children under age two is best supervised by a knowledgeable herbalist. The child's doctor should be consulted or informed of herbal treatments as well. Consult with a lactation specialist before feeding any herbal preparations to an exclusively breastfed infant. Consider external forms of herbal treatment, such as baths or massage. For many herbs, nursing mothers can take the herb and provide benefit to the breastfeeding child (see chapter 10).

The Plant Safety Table
The following ratings are drawn mainly from *American Herbal Products Association's Botanical Safety Handbook,* by McGuffin, et al. (1997); *Botanical Medicines: The Desk Reference for Major Herbal Supplements,* 2nd edition, by D. McKenna, et al. (2002); *The Complete German Commission E Monographs,* edited by Blumenthal, et al. (1998); *Handbook of Medicinal Herbs,* 1st and 2nd editions, by James Duke (1985, 2002); *Herbal Drugs and Phytopharmaceuticals,* English edition (referred to as "Teedrogen"), edited by Norman Grainger Bisset and Max Wichtl (2001); *Phytotherapy in Paediatrics,* by H. Schilcher (1997); *Potter's New Cyclopaedia of Botanical Drugs and Preparations* (referred to as "Potter"), by R. C. Wren, revised by Elizabeth M. Williamson and Fred J. Evans (1988); and *Principles and Practice of Phytotherapy,* by S. Mills and K. Bone (1999). See appendix A for more information on these reference texts.

Common Name	Botanical Name	Part Used	Safety Rating	Notes
adzuki bean	*Vigna angularis*	seed	A	galactogogue
agastache	*Agastache rugosa*	leaf, stem	A	
alder buckthorn	*Rhamnus frangula*	bark	C	
alfalfa	*Medicago sativa*	blooming plant (flower, leaf, stem), seed	A, plant; C, seed	galactogogue
alkanet	*Alkanna tinctoria*	root	C	
allspice	*Pimenta dioica*	unripe fruit	A	
aloe vera gel	*Aloe vera*	interior leaf	B	do not use on nipples
aloes	*Aloe ferox, A. perryi, A. vera, A. barbadensis*	leaf skin latex	C	
American hellebore	*Veratrum viride*	fruit	E	
American mistletoe	*Phoradendron leucarpum*	leaf, stem	E	
angelica	*Angelica archangelica, A. purpurea, A. pubescens*	seed, root, leaf, stem	B	photosensitizing
anise	*Pimpinella anisum*	seed	B	galactogogue; allergenic (occasional)
annatto	*Bixa orellana*	seed	A	
apricot seed	*Prunus armeniaca*	seed	C	
aristolochia	*Aristolochia* species	leaf, stem, rhizome, fruit	E	

Common Name	Botanical Name	Part Used	Safety Rating	Notes
arnica	*Arnica latifolia, A. montana,* and other *Arnica* species	leaf, stem, infusion oil	C, external; E, internal	contact allergen; do not use on nipples
arrow poison	*Strophanthus* species *(S. kombé, S. gratus, S. hisbidus, S. sarmentosus, S. gardeniiflorus)*	seed	E	all species are poisonous
arrowroot	*Maranta arundinacea*	root	A	
artichoke	*Cynara cardunculus* subspecies *cardunculus*	blooming plant (flower, leaf, stem)	A	contact allergen (occasional)
asarabacca	*Asarum europaeum*	leaf, stem, rhizome	C	
ashwagandha	*Withania somnifera*	root	C	galactogogue
asparagus	*Asparagus officinalis*	root	C	contact allergen (rare)
astragalus	*Astragalus membranaceus, A. mongholicus*	root	A	
autumn crocus	*Colchicum autumnale*	flower, seed, tuber	D	contains colchicine, which requires supervision by a physician and lactation consultant
avocado	*Persea americana*	fruit pulp	A	
bai he	*Lilium brownii*	bulb	A	
bai wei	*Cynanchum atratum*	root	A	

Common Name	Botanical Name	Part Used	Safety Rating	Notes
bai zhu	*Atractylodes macrocephala*	rhizome	A	
balmony	*Chelone glabra*	leaf, stem, flower	A	
balsam fir	*Abies balsamea*	bark	A	
banana	*Musa x paradisiaca*	leaf, flower bud	B	galactogogue
barberry	*Berberis vulgaris*	root, root bark	C	
barley	*Hordeum vulgare*	green shoot, seed	A	galactogogue
barley sprout	*Hordeum vulgare*	sprout (fried)	A	antigalactogogue
basil	*Ocimum basilicum*	leaf, stem	B	
bay leaf	*Laurus nobilis*	leaf	A	contact allergen
belladonna	*Atropa belladonna*	leaf	D	contains atropine alkaloids, which require supervision by a physician and lactation consultant
benzoin	*Styrax benzoin, S. paralleloneurum, S. tonkinensis*	gum resin	A	
bergamot orange	*Citrus bergamia*	peel	A	potential allergen
bilberry	*Vaccinium myrtillus*	fruit, leaf	A, fruit; C, leaf	insufficient data to determine the safety of the leaf

Common Name	Botanical Name	Part Used	Safety Rating	Notes
birch	*Betula* species	leaf, bark	B	bark is allergenic
birthroot (beth root)	*Trillium erectum*	root	B	endangered
bishop's weed	*Amni visnaga*	fruit	C	photosensitizing, allergenic
bistort	*Polygonum bistorta*	root	A	
bitter almond	*Prunus dulcis* var. *amara*	seed	C	
bitter apple	*Citrullus colocynthis*	fruit	E	
bitter melon	*Momordica charantia*	leaf	C	galactogogue
bitter orange	*Citrus aurantium*	fruit peel	B	allergenic; stimulant
black cohosh	*Actaea racemosa* (*Cimicifuga racemosa*)	rhizome	B	galactogogue; allergenic
black cumin	*Nigella sativa*	seed	A	galactogogue
black currant	*Ribes nigrum* var. *chlorocarpum*	fruit, seed oil	A	
black haw	*Viburnum prunifolium*	bark	B	
black hellebore	*Helleborus niger*	rhizome	E	
black horehound	*Ballota nigra*	leaf, stem	B	
black mulberry	*Morus nigra*	fruit	A	
black pepper	*Piper nigrum*	fruit	A	galactogogue
black tea	*Camellia sinensis*	fermented leaf	B	galactogogue; stimulant (caffeine)

Common Name	Botanical Name	Part Used	Safety Rating	Notes
black walnut	*Juglans nigra*	hull, leaf	C	
bladder wrack	*Fucus vesiculosus, Fucus* species	seaweed thallus	B	allergenic; contains iodine
blessed thistle	*Cnicus benedictus*	leaf, stem, flower	B	galactogogue; allergenic (rare)
bloodroot	*Sanguinaria canadensis*	root	C	endangered
blue cohosh	*Caulophyllum thalictroides*	root	C	endangered
blue flag	*Iris versicolor, I. virginica*	rhizome, root	C	
blueberry	*Vaccinium angustifolium, V. corymbosum V. pallidum*	leaf, fruit	A	
bogbean	*Menyanthes trifoliata*	leaf	B	
boldo	*Peumus boldus*	leaf, bark	B	
boneset	*Eupatorium perfoliatum*	leaf, stem	C	
borage	*Borago officinalis*	leaf, flower	C	galactogogue; leaf contains tiny amounts of toxic pyrrolizidine alkaloids
borage seed oil	*Borago officinalis*	pressed seed oil	A	galactogogue?
boxwood	*Buxus sempervirens*	leaf	E	
brahmi	*Bacopa monnieri*	leaf, stem	B	

Common Name	Botanical Name	Part Used	Safety Rating	Notes
Brazil nut	*Bertholletia excelsa*	nut	A	allergenic
Brazilian rosewood	*Aniba rosaeodora*	bark	A	
British elecampane (xuan fu hua)	*Inula britannica*	flower	A	photosensitizing
broomrape	*Cistanche salsa*	root	A	
brown rice	*Oryza sativa*	seed	A	galactogogue
bryony	*Bryonia* species	root	E	
buchu	*Agathosma betulina*	leaf	C	
buckwheat	*Fagopyrum esculentum*	blooming plant (flower, leaf, stem)	A	seed is allergenic
bugleweed	*Lycopus europaeus, L. americanus, L. virginicus*	leaf, stem	C	antigalactogogue
burdock	*Arctium lappa*	root	B	contact allergen
butcher's broom	*Ruscus aculeatus*	root	A	
butterbur	*Petasites* species	leaf, root	E	
butterfly weed	*Asclepias tuberosa*	root	C	
butternut	*Juglans cineraria*	root bark	C	
cabbage	*Brassica oleracea* var. *capitata*	leaf	A	external antigalactogogue

Common Name	Botanical Name	Part Used	Safety Rating	Notes
Calabar bean	*Physostigma venenosum*	ripe seed	E	
calendula	*Calendula officinalis*	flower	A	
camphor	*Cinnamomum camphora*	distillate of wood	C	allergenic; do not use on or near infant's face, especially the nose
camu-camu	*Myrciaria dubia*	fruit	A	
Canada fleabane	*Conyza canadensis*	leaf, stem	A	
cang zhu	*Atractylodes lancea*	rhizome	A	
cao guo	*Amomum tsao-ko*	fruit	A	
caper	*Physalis peruviana*	fruit	A	
caraway	*Carum carvi*	seed, essential oil	A	galactogogue
cardamom	*Elettaria cardamomum*	fruit	A	
carob	*Ceratonia siliqua*	fruit	A	
cascara sagrada	*Rhamnus purshiana*	bark	B	
cashew	*Anacardium occidentale*	nut	A	allergenic
castor oil	*Ricinus communis*	seed oil, leaf	C	leaf is a galactogogue (safety unknown); seed is toxic
catnip	*Nepeta* species	leaf, stem	B	
cat's claw	*Uncaria tomentosa*	root, root bark	C	galactogogue?; photosensitizing
catuaba	*Erythroxylum catuaba*	bark	E	

Common Name	Botanical Name	Part Used	Safety Rating	Notes
cayenne	*Capsicum annuum*	fruit	B	
celandine	*Chelidonium majus*	leaf, stem	B	
celery	*Apium graveolens*	seed	C	galactogogue; all parts photosensitizing, allergenic
centaury	*Centaurium erythraea*	blooming plant (flower, leaf, stem)	A	
chai hu	*Bupleurum chinensis* and other species	root	A	
chamomile	*Matricaria recutita*	blooming plant (flower, leaf, stem)	A/B	allergenic (rare)
chaparral	*Larrea tridentata*	leaf, stem	E	insufficient data
chapeau de couro	*Echinodorus macrophyllus*	leaf, bark, root	A	
chasteberry	*Vitex agnus-castus*	fruit, leaf	B	studies have shown both galactogogue and antigalactogogue activity; allergenic
chia	*Salvia columbariae*	seed	A	
chickweed	*Stellaria media*	leaf, stem	A	galactogogue
chicory	*Chicorium intybus*	leaf, stem, root	A	allergenic
Chinaberry	*Melia azedarach*	root, root bark	E	

Common Name	Botanical Name	Part Used	Safety Rating	Notes
Chinese asparagus	*Asparagus cochinchinensis*	processed rhizome	A	
Chinese peony	*Paeonia lactiflora*	root	A	
Chinese rhubarb	*Rheum palmatum, R. officinale,* and other *Rheum* species	rhizome	C	garden rhubarb stalks used as food
Chinese yam	*Dioscorea opposita*	root	A	
chive	*Allium schoenoprasum*	leaf	A	
chocolate (cocoa)	*Theobroma cacao*	bean	B	allergenic; stimulant for some babies
chocolate vine	*Akebia quinata*	leaf	B	galactogogue
cinchona	*Cinchona pubescens* and other *Cinchona* species	bark	C	allergenic
cinnamon	*Cinnamomum aromaticum, C. verum*	flower, bark	B	allergenic
clary sage	*Salvia sclarea*	leaf, stem	A	
cleavers	*Galium aparine, G. verum*	leaf, stem	A	
clove	*Syzygium aromaticum*	bud	A	
clubmoss	*Lycopodium clavatum*	plant, spore	C	
coconut	*Cocos nucifera*	seed milk	A	galactogogue
codonopsis	*Codonopsis pilosula, C. tangshen*	root	A	

Common Name	Botanical Name	Part Used	Safety Rating	Notes
coffee	*Coffea arabica*	bean	B	galactogogue; stimulant (caffeine)
cola	*Cola acuminata, C. nitida*	seed	B	mild stimulant
collinsonia	*Collinsonia canadensis*	root	A	
coltsfoot	*Tussilago farfara*	leaf, flower	E	
comfrey leaf	*Symphytum officinale*	leaf	B, external; C, internal	leaf products labeled "< 1 ppm pyrrolizidine alkaloids" are safer
comfrey root	*Symphytum officinale*	root	C, external; E, internal	root products labeled "< 1 ppm pyrrolizidine alkaloids" are safer
condurango	*Marsdenia condurango*	bark	C	
cordyceps	*Cordyceps sinensis*	fruiting body	A	
coriander (cilantro)	*Coriandrum sativum*	seed, young shoot	A	seed is galactogogue
corn ergot	*Ustilago zeae*	fungus	E	
cornflower	*Centaurea cyanus*	leaf, stem	A	
corn silk	*Zea mays*	stigma	A	
cotton seed	*Gossypium* species	seed	C	galactogogue
couch grass	*Elytrigia repens*	rhizome	A	
cowslip	*Primula veris*	root	A	allergenic

Common Name	Botanical Name	Part Used	Safety Rating	Notes
cramp bark	*Viburnum opulus*	root bark	A	
cranberry	*Vaccinium macrocarpum*	fruit	A	
cranesbill	*Geranium maculatum*	root	A	
cumin	*Cuminum cyminum*	seed	A	galactogogue
damiana	*Turnera diffusa* var. *diffusa*	leaf	B	
dandelion	*Taraxacum officinalis*	leaf, flower, rhizome	A, leaf, flower; B, rhizome	galactogogue; allergenic (rare)
dead nettle	*Lamium album*	leaf, stem	A	
devil's claw	*Harpagophytum procumben*	tuber	C	galactogogue?; allergenic
devil's club	*Oplopanax horridus*	root	A	
dill	*Anethum graveolens*	seed, essential oil	A	galactogogue
dodder	*Cuscuta chinensis, C. japonica*	seed	A	
dong quai	*Angelica sinensis*	rhizome	B	
dulse	*Rhodymenia palmata*	thallus	B	
dusty miller	*Senecio cineraria*	leaf, stem, flower	E	
dyer's broom	*Genista tinctoria*	leaf, stem, flower	C	

Common Name	Botanical Name	Part Used	Safety Rating	Notes
Eastern red cedar	*Juniperus virginiana*	leaf, berry	E	
Eastern white cedar	*Thuja occidentalis*	stem, frond	C	
echinacea	*Echinacea angustifolia, E. pallida, E. purpurea*	stem, leaf, flower, root	B	
elecampane	*Inula helenium*	rhizome, root	C	strongly allergenic
eleuthero (Siberian ginseng)	*Eleutherococcus senticosus*	rhizome	B	
emblic	*Phyllanthus emblica*	fruit	A	
ephedra (ma huang)	*Ephedra sinica* and other *Ephedra* species (except *E. nevadensis*)	stem	C	antigalactogogue; stimulant
ergot	*Claviceps purpurea*	fungus	E	
erythrina	*Erythrina variegata* var. *orientalis*	bark	A	galactogogue
eucalyptus	*Eucalyptus globulus*	leaf, essential oil	B, external; E, internal (oil)	do not use oil on or near baby's face, especially the nose
eucommia	*Eucommia ulmoides*	bark	A	
European corn mint	*Mentha arvensis*	leaf, essential oil	A	antigalactogogue?; do not use oil on or near baby's face, especially the nose
European elder	*Sambucus nigra*	flower, ripened fruit	A	flower is a galactogogue

Common Name	Botanical Name	Part Used	Safety Rating	Notes
European hazelnut	*Corylus avellana, C. cornuta*	leaf, bark	A	
European mistletoe	*Viscum album*	leaf, stem, fruit	C	allergenic
European peony	*Paeonia officinalis*	root	A	
European sanicle	*Sanicula europaea*	leaf, stem	A	
evening primrose	*Oenothera biennis*	seed oil, leaf, stem	A	
eyebright	*Euphrasia officinalis*	leaf, stem	A	endangered
false hellebore	*Adonis vernalis*	leaf, stem	C	
false unicorn	*Chamaelirium luteum*	rhizome	B	endangered
fang feng	*Ledebouriella seseloides*	root	A	
fang ji (Stephania)	*Stephania tetrandra*	root	C	may be adulterated with toxic plant, *Aristolochia fangchi*
fava bean	*Vicia faba*	flower, well-cooked bean	B	antigalactogogue?; sensitivity reaction (favism)
fennel	*Foeniculum vulgare*	seed, essential oil	A, seed; B, essential oil	galactogogue; allergenic (very rare)
fenugreek	*Trigonella foenum-graecum*	seed	B	galactogogue; allergenic
feverfew	*Tanacetum parthenium*	leaf	B	allergenic

Common Name	Botanical Name	Part Used	Safety Rating	Notes
fig	*Ficus carica*	green fruit	A	galactogogue
fir needles	*Picea abies, Abies alba,* and other *Abies* species	essential oil	B	allergenic
flannelweed	*Sida cordifolia*	flower, leaf	C	antigalactogogue?; stimulant
flax	*Linum usitatissimum*	ripe seed, fresh oil	B	allergenic
fo–ti	*Polygonum multiflorum*	dry root	B	allergenic
foxglove	*Digitalis* species	leaf	D	contains digitoxin and digoxin, which require supervision by a physician and lactation consultant
frankincense	*Boswellia carteri, B. serrata*	gum resin	A	
fringetree	*Chionanthus virginicus*	root	A	
fu ling	*Wolfiporia cocos*	sclerotium	A	
gao ben	*Ligusticum sinense*	root, rhizome	A	
garden cress	*Lepidium sativum*	seed	B	galactogogue
garlic	*Allium sativum*	bulb	B	galactogogue; allergenic
germander	*Teucrium chamaedrys* and other *Teucrium* species	leaf, stem	E	common contaminant of skullcap products
ginger	*Zingiber officinale*	root	B	fresh root is a galactogogue

Common Name	Botanical Name	Part Used	Safety Rating	Notes
ginkgo	*Ginkgo biloba*	leaf extract	B	allergenic
ginseng	*Panax ginseng, P. quinquefolia*	rhizome	B	
glehnia	*Glehnia littoralis*	root	A	
glossy privet	*Ligusticum lucidum*	fruit	A	
goat's rue	*Galega officinalis*	blooming plant (flower, leaf, stem)	B	galactogogue; use dried herb or tincture
golden-eye grass	*Curculigo orchioides*	rhizome	C	
goldenseal	*Hydrastis canadensis*	rhizome, root	C	endangered
gotu cola	*Centella asiatica*	leaf, stem	B	allergenic
gou ji	*Cibotium barometz*	rhizome	A	
grains of paradise	*Amomum melegueta*	fruit, seed	A	
grape	*Vitis vinifera*	fruit, leaf, seed extract	A	seed is allergenic
grapefruit seed extract	*Citrus* x *paradisi* and other *Citrus* species	seed	A	allergenic
greater galangal (ka or laos)	*Alpinia galanga*	rhizome	A	
Greek oregano	*Salvia fruticosa*	leaf	A	antigalactogogue?
green tea	*Camellia sinensis*	leaf	B	galactogogue; mild stimulant (caffeine)
ground ivy	*Glechoma hederacea*	leaf, stem	B	

Common Name	Botanical Name	Part Used	Safety Rating	Notes
groundsel	*Senecio vulgaris*	leaf, stem	E	
gu sui bu	*Drynaria fortunei*	rhizome	A	
guang fang ji	*Aristolochia fangchi*	leaf, stem	E	
guarana	*Paullinia cupana*	seed	B	stimulant (caffeine)
guggul	*Commiphora mukul*	gum resin	B	
gum arabic	*Acacia senegal*	gum resin	A	
gymnema	*Gymnema sylvestre*	leaf	C	galactogogue
han lian cao	*Eclipta prostrata*	leaf, stem	A	
hawthorn	*Crataegus* species	leaf, flower, fruit	B	
hay flower	various species of the *Poaceae* (grass) family	leaf, stem	B	external use contact allergenic (rare)
he huan pi	*Albizia julibrissin*	flower	A	
heal-all	*Prunella vulgaris*	leaf, stem	A	
heartsease	*Viola tricolor*	leaf, stem	A	
heather	*Calluna vulgaris*	flower	A	
hemp-agrimony	*Eupatorium cannabinum*	leaf, stem	E	
henbane	*Hyoscyamus niger*	blooming plant (flower, leaf, stem)	D	contains atropine alkaloids, which require supervision by a physician and lactation consultant

Common Name	Botanical Name	Part Used	Safety Rating	Notes
henna	*Lawsonia inermis*	leaf	C	external use only
hibiscus	*Hibiscus* species	flower	A	galactogogue
high mallow	*Malva sylvestris*	leaf, flower	A	
hollyhock	*Alcea rosea*	root	A	
holy basil	*Ocimum tenuiflorum (O. sanctum)*	leaf	B	antigalactogogue?
hops	*Humulus lupulus*	strobilus	B	galactogogue; contact allergenic
horehound	*Marrubium vulgare*	leaf, stem	B	
horse chestnut	*Aesculus hippocastanum*	seed	B	
horsetail	*Equisetum arvense*	shoot	C	
hound's-tongue	*Cynoglossum officinale*	leaf, stem	E	
huang jing	*Polygonatum sibericum*	root	A	
hyssop	*Hyssopus officinalis*	blooming plant (flower, leaf, stem)	B, herb; E, essential oil	
Iceland moss	*Cetraria islandica*	lichen thallus	B	galactogogue; allergenic (rare)
Indian coral tree	*Erythrina variegata*	leaf	C	galactogogue
Indian elecampane	*Inula racemosa*	root	C	allergenic
Indian sarsaparilla	*Hemidesmus indicus*	root	E	

Common Name	Botanical Name	Part Used	Safety Rating	Notes
Indian snakeroot	*Rauwolfia* species	root	D	galactogogue; contains reserpine, which requires supervision by a physician and lactation consultant
ipecac	*Cephaelis ipecacuanha*	root, rhizome	C	
ixbut	*Euphorbia lancifolia*	leaf	C	galactogogue
jaborandi	*Pilocarpus jaborandi* and other *Pilocarpus* species	leaflet	D	galactogogue; contains pilocarpine, which requires supervision by a physician and lactation consultant
jalap	*Ipomoea purga*	tuberous root	E	
Jamaican dogwood	*Piscidia erythrina*	root bark	C	
jambolan plum	*Syzygium cumini*	bark, seed, root	A	root is a galactogogue
Japanese apricot	*Prunus mume*	unripe fruit	A	
Japanese honeysuckle	*Lonicera japonica*	flowers, stem	A	
jasmine	*Jasminum sambac*	flower	B	external antigalactogogue
Jerusalem artichoke	*Helianthus tuberosus*	tuber	A	galactogogue
jimson weed	*Datura* species	leaf, stem	E	
jin yin hua	*Lonicera japonica*	flower	A	

Common Name	Botanical Name	Part Used	Safety Rating	Notes
jivanti	*Leptadenia reticulata*	seed	C	galactogogue; limited information
joe-pye weed	*Eupatorium purpureum*	rhizome, root	E	
jujube	*Ziziphus jujuba*	fruit	A	
juniper	*Juniperus communis, J. oxycedrus*	fruit	B	
jute	*Corchorus olitorius*	leaf	A	
kava	*Piper methysticum*	rhizome	C	allergenic
kelp	general term for large brown algae, e.g. *Laminaria hyperborea*	seaweed thallus	B	allergenic; contains iodine
kudzu	*Pueraria lobata, P. thomsonii*	leaf, stem, root	A	galactogogue
lady's mantle	*Alchemilla xanthochlora*	leaf	B	galactogogue
lamb's quarters	*Chenopodium album*	leaf, stem	B	galactogogue
larch turpentine	*Larix decidua*	resin	B	allergenic
large-leafed linden	*Tilia platyphyllos*	leaf, flower	A	
lavender	*Lavandula* species	flower	A	galactogogue; allergenic (very rare)
lemon	*Citrus limon*	peel	A	allergenic
lemon balm	*Melissa officinalis*	leaf	A	galactogogue?
lemon thyme	*Thymus* x *citriodorus*	leaf	A	
lemon verbena	*Aloysia triphylla*	leaf	A	

Common Name	Botanical Name	Part Used	Safety Rating	Notes
lemongrass	*Cymbopogon citratus*	leaf, stem	A	
lesser galangal (kencur or krachai)	*Alpinia officinarum*	rhizome	A	
licorice	*Glycyrrhiza glabra* and other *Glycyrrhiza* species	rhizome	B	galactogogue
life root	*Senecio aureus*	leaf, stem	E	
lily of the valley	*Convallaria majalis*	leaf, stem	C	
lime	*Citrus aurantifolia*	peel	A	allergenic
linden	*Tilia* x *europaea*	leaf, flower	A	
lobelia	*Lobelia inflata*	leaf, stem	C	
long birthwort	*Aristolochia clematitis*	leaf, stem, rhizome	E	
long pepper	*Piper longum*	fruit	A	galactogogue
longan	*Dimocarpus longan*	fruit	A	
loquat	*Eriobotrya japonica*	leaf	C	
ma dou ling (qing mu xiang or tian zian teng)	*Aristolochia* species	fruit	E	
Madagascar periwinkle	*Catharanthus roseus*	leaf, stem, root, flower	E	
madder	*Rubia tinctorum*	root	E	
magnolia	*Magnolia officinalis*	flower, bark	A, flower; B, bark	

Common Name	Botanical Name	Part Used	Safety Rating	Notes
mai dong	*Ophiopogon japonicus*	root	A	
maidenhair fern	*Adiantum pedatum*	leaf, stem	B	
maitake	*Grifola frondosa*	fruiting body, mycelium	A	
male fern	*Dryopteris filix-mas*	rhizome	E	
mandarin orange	*Citrus reticulata*	peel	A	allergenic
mandrake	*Mandragora officinarum*	root	E	
mango	*Mangifera indica*	fruit skin	A	allergenic
mao gen	*Imperata cylindrica*	rhizome	A	
marsh tea	*Ledum palustre*	leaf	C	
marshmallow	*Althaea officinalis*	root	A	galactogogue
mayapple	*Podophyllum peltatum*	root, resin	C, external; E, internal	
mei gui hua	*Rosa rugosa*	flower	A	
mesquite	*Prosopis juliflora*	pollen, fruit	A	allergenic
Mexican bamboo	*Fallopia japonica*	shoot, dry root	A	
milk thistle	*Silybum marianum*	seed, stem	A	galactogogue
Missouri snakeroot	*Parthenium integrifolium*	root	A	

Common Name	Botanical Name	Part Used	Safety Rating	Notes
monkshood	*Aconitum napellus* and other *Aconitum* species	root, tuber	E	
moringa	*Moringa oleifera*	fruit, bark	B	fruit is a galactogogue
Mormon tea	*Ephedra nevadensis*	leaf, stem	A	
mother of thyme	*Thymus serpyllum*	leaf, stem	B	essential oil is toxic, allergenic
motherwort	*Leonurus cardiaca*	leaf, stem	B	photosensitizing
mu xiang	*Saussurea lappa*	root	A	
mugwort	*Artemisia vulgaris*	leaf, stem, flower, essential oil	B	antigalactogogue; allergenic
muira puama	*Ptychopetalum olacoides, P. uncinatum*	wood, root	A	
mullein	*Verbascum thapsus, V. densiflorum, V. phlomoides*	leaf, flower	A	
mum	*Chrysanthemum* x *morifolium*	flower	A	allergenic
mung bean	*Vigna radiata*	seed	A	galactogogue
myrrh	*Commiphora myrrha, C. madagascariensis, C. molmol*	gum resin	B	
New Zealand spinach	*Basella alba*	leaf	A	galactogogue
noni	*Morinda citrifolia*	fruit, leaf	A	

Common Name	Botanical Name	Part Used	Safety Rating	Notes
nut grass	*Cyperus rotundus*	tuber	A	galactogogue
nutmeg	*Myristica fragrans*	seed, essential oil	C	
nux vomica	*Strychnos nux-vomica*	seed	E	
oak	*Quercus alba*	bark	B	
oats	*Avena sativa*	seed, straw	A	galactogogue
okra	*Abelmoschus esculentus*	fruit	A	galactogogue
oleander	*Nerium oleander*	leaf	E	
olive	*Olea europaea*	leaf	A	galactogogue
onion	*Allium cepa*	bulb	A	allergenic
Oregon grape	*Mahonia* species	root	C	
oriental arborvitae (bai zi ren)	*Platycladus orientalis*	seed, leafy twig	A, seed; C, leafy twig	
osha	*Ligusticum porteri*	root	B	antigalactogogue; endangered
papaya	*Carica papaya*	green fruit, leaf	B	galactogogue; allergenic
parsley	*Petroselinum crispum*	leaf, stem	B	antigalactogogue (in large amounts); allergenic
parsley seed	*Petroselinum crispum*	seed, essential oil	E	
partridge berry	*Mitchella repens*	leaf, stem	A	galactogogue

Common Name	Botanical Name	Part Used	Safety Rating	Notes
passionflower	*Passiflora incarnata*	leaf, stem	A	
patchouli	*Pogostemon cablin*	leaf, stem	B	
pea	*Pisum sativum*	seed	A	galactogogue
peach	*Prunus persica*	seed, leaf	C	
peanut	*Arachis hypogaea*	seed	A	galactogogue; allergenic
pearly everlasting	*Anaphalis margaritacea*	leaf, stem	A	
pedra hume caa	*Myrcia sphaerocarpa*	leaf, stem	A	
pellitory of the wall	*Parietaria judaica, P. officinalis*	leaf, stem	A	
pennyroyal	*Hedeoma pulegioides (Mentha pulegium)*	leaf, essential oil	C, leaf; E, essential oil	essential oil is toxic
peppermint	*Mentha x piperita*	leaf, essential oil	A, leaf; B, essential oil	essential oil is an antigalactogogue; do not use on or near baby's face, especially the nose
periwinkle	*Vinca minor*	leaf, stem	B	antigalactogogue
Peruvian balsam	*Myroxylon balsamum* var. *pereira*	resin	C	external use only; allergenic (contains bromelain)
pfaffia	*Pfaffia paniculata*	root	A	

Common Name	Botanical Name	Part Used	Safety Rating	Notes
pigeon pea	*Cajanus cajan*	pod, seed, leaf	A	antigalactogogue
pill-bearing spurge	*Euphorbia pilulifera*	leaf, stem	C	allergenic
pine needle	*Pinus sylvestris* and other *Pinus* species	leaf essential oil	A	allergenic
pineapple	*Ananas comosus*	fruit	A	allergenic
pineapple weed	*Chamomilla suaveolens*	blooming plant (leaf, stem, flower)	A	galactogogue?
pink peppercorn	*Schinus* species	bark, fruit	B	
plantain	*Plantago major*	leaf	B	galactogogue
poison hemlock	*Conium maculatum*	seed	E	
poke (pokeweed)	*Phytolacca americana*	root, leaf, fruit	C/E	toxicity varies with maturity of plant
pollen	various species	raw flower pollen	A	allergenic
pomegranate	*Punica granatum*	stem bark, root, root bark	E	
poplar	*Populus* species	bud	A	allergenic
potato	*Solanum tuberosum*	tuber	A	galactogogue
premna	*Premna obtusifolia*	leaf, root	B	galactogogue
prickly ash	*Zanthoxylum americanum*, *Z. clava-herculis*	bark, fruit	C	

Common Name	Botanical Name	Part Used	Safety Rating	Notes
psyllium	*Plantago psyllium, P. ovata*	seed, husk	A	allergenic
pulsatilla	*Anemone pulsatilla*	leaf, stem	C	
pumpkin	*Cucurbita pepo*	seed	A	
purging buckthorn	*Rhamnus catharticus*	fruit	C	
purging croton	*Croton tiglium*	seed, seed oil	E	
purslane	*Portulaca oleracea*	leaf	B	galactogogue
pygeum	*Prunus africana*	leaf	A	antigalactogogue
qian shi	*Euryale ferox*	seed	A	
qiang huo	*Notopterygium incisum*	rhizome	A	
qing guo	*Canarium album*	fruit	A	
quebracho	*Aspidosperma quebracho-blanco*	bark	B	
queen's delight	*Stillingia sylvatica*	dried root	C	avoid when nursing
quillaja	*Quillaja saponaria*	bark	C	
radish	*Raphanus sativus*	seed	B	galactogogue
ragwort	*Senecio jacobaea*	leaf, stem	E	
ramson	*Allium ursinum*	root, shoot	A	allergenic
raspberry	*Rubus idaeus*	leaf	A	galactogogue
red clover	*Trifolium pratense*	leaf, stem, flower	B	galactogogue

Common Name	Botanical Name	Part Used	Safety Rating	Notes
red currant	*Ribes rubrum*	fruit, leaf	A	
red magnolia	*Magnolia liliflora*	flower	A	
red mulberry	*Morus rubra*	fruit, leaf	A	
red sandalwood	*Pterocarpus santalinus*	heartwood	A	
reishi	*Ganoderma lucidum*	mushroom thallus	B	allergenic
rhatany	*Krameria triandra, K. argentea*	root	C	allergenic
rhodiola	*Rhodiola rosea*	root	B	
Roman chamomile	*Chamaemelum nobile*	flower	A	allergenic
rooibos	*Aspalathus* species	leaf	A	
rose geranium	*Pelargonium graveolens*	leaf	A	galactogogue?
rose hips	*Rosa* species	fruit	A	
rosemary	*Rosmarinus officinalis*	leaf	B	antigalactogogue?
rue	*Ruta graveolens*	leaf, stem	C	allergenic
Russian comfrey	*Symphytum asperum, Symphytum x uplandicum,* and other cultivars	root, leaf	E	
sage	*Salvia officinalis*	leaf	B	antigalactogogue
sassafras	*Sassafras albidum*	leaf, root bark, filé	C	

Common Name	Botanical Name	Part Used	Safety Rating	Notes
saw palmetto	*Serenoa repens*	fruit	A	
sawbrier	*Smilax glauca*	root	A	
scammony	*Convolvulus scammonia*	root, root resin	E	
scopolia	*Scopolia carniolica*	rhizome	D	contains atropine alkaloids, which require supervision by a physician and lactation consultant
Scotch broom	*Cytisus scoparius*	blooming plant (leaf, stem, flower)	C	
sea holly	*Eryngium maritimum, E. planum, E. yuccifolium*	root	A	
senecio	*Senecio* species	leaf, stem	E	
senna	*Senna alexandrina, S. obtusifolia, S. tora; Cassia* species	leaf, fruit	B	
sesame	*Sesamum indicum, S. orientale*	seed	A	galactogogue; allergenic
shakuyaku-kanzo-to (peony and licorice)	*Paeonia officinalis* and *Glycyrrhiza* species in combination	rhizome	B	antigalactogogue
shatavari	*Asparagus racemosa*	root	B	galactogogue
she chuang zi	*Cnidium monnieri*	seed	A	

Common Name	Botanical Name	Part Used	Safety Rating	Notes
shepherd's purse	*Capsella bursa-pastoris*	leaf, stem	B	
shiitake	*Lentinus edodes*	fruiting body, mycelium	A	
skullcap	*Scutellaria lateriflora*	leaf, stem	B	some skullcap products are contaminated with germander (safety rating: E)
skunk cabbage	*Symplocarpus foetidus*	dried rhizome and root	C	
slippery elm	*Ulmus rubra*	bark	A	endangered
sloe	*Prunus spinosa*	seed, fresh flower	B	
Solomon's seal	*Polygonatum biflorum*	root	A	
sorrel	*Rumex acetosa, R. acetosella*	leaf	B	
soybean	*Glycine max*	seed	A	
spearmint	*Mentha spicata*	leaf	A	
speedwell	*Veronica officinalis*	leaf, stem	A	
spreading dogbane	*Apocynum androsaemifolium*	root	E	
squill	*Drimia maritima (Urginea maritima)*	bulb	C	

Common Name	Botanical Name	Part Used	Safety Rating	Notes
St. John's wort	*Hypericum perforatum*	infusion oil, blooming plant (leaf, stem, flower)	B	galactogogue?; allergenic
star anise	*Illicium verum*	fruit	C	galactogogue; allergenic; potential toxicity from product contamination
stevia	*Stevia rebaudiana*	leaf	A	
stinging nettle	*Urtica dioica, U. urens*	leaf, stem, flower	A	galactogogue
strawberry	*Fragaria vesca, F. virginiana*	leaf	A	
sumac	*Rhus coriaria, R. glabra*	fruit	A	
sunflower	*Helianthus annuus*	seed	A	
Surinam cherry	*Eugenia uniflora*	fruit	A	
sweet annie	*Artemisia annua*	leaf, stem	A	allergenic
sweet bay	*Magnolia virginiana*	bark	A	
sweet cicely	*Myrrhis odorata*	fruit, leaf, stem, root	A	galactogogue; allergenic (rare)
sweet flag	*Acorus calamus,* four varieties	rhizome	C	
sweet marjoram	*Origanum majorana*	leaf	A	galactogogue?
sweet potato	*Ipomoea batatas*	tuber	A	galactogogue
sweet violet	*Viola odorata*	leaf	A	

Common Name	Botanical Name	Part Used	Safety Rating	Notes
tamarind	*Tamarindus indica*	fruit	A	galactogogue
tansy	*Tanacetum vulgare*	leaf, stem	C	
taro	*Colocasia esculenta*	root	A	galactogogue
tarragon (French tarragon)	*Artemisia dracunculus*	essential oil	C	
tea tree oil	*Melaleuca alternifolia*	essential oil	C, external; E, internal	contact allergen; do not use essential oil on or near baby's face, especially the nose
teasel	*Dipsacus asper, D. japonicus*	root	A	
tian ma	*Gastrodia elata*	rhizome	A	
tolu balsam	*Myroxylon balsamum* var. *balsamum*	resin	B	
tonka bean	*Dipteryx odorata, D. oppositifolia*	seed	C	
toothache plant	*Spilanthes acmella, S. oleracea*	leaf, stem	A	galactogogue
tragacanth	*Astragalus gummifer*	fruit	A	
tree moss	*Evernia* species	thallus	C	
trichosanthes	*Trichosanthes kirilowii*	fruit, seed, root	A, fruit, seed; B, root	
turmeric	*Curcuma domestica, C. longa*	rhizome	B	galactogogue

Common Name	Botanical Name	Part Used	Safety Rating	Notes
usnea	*Usnea barbata* and other *Usnea* species	lichen thallus	A	
uva-ursi	*Arctostaphylos uva-ursi*	leaf	C	antigalactogogue?
valerian	*Valeriana officinalis*	root, rhizome	A	
vanilla	*Vanilla planifolia, V. tahitensis*	fruit	A	
velvet bean	*Mucuna pruriens*	pod hair, seed	C	antigalactogogue?
vervain	*Verbena officinalis*	blooming plant (flower, leaf, stem)	B	galactogogue
vetiver	*Vetiveria zizanioides*	root	C	
viper's bugloss	*Echium vulgare*	seed	E	galactogogue
Virginia snakeroot	*Aristolochia serpentaria*	rhizome	E	
wahoo	*Euonymus atropurpureus*	root bark	C	
walnut	*Juglans regia*	hull, leaf	C	
water mint	*Mentha aquatica* var. *glabrata*	leaf	A	antigalactogogue?
watercress	*Nasturtium officinale*	leaf	B	
wax gourd	*Benincasa hispida*	rind	A	
white ash	*Fraxinus americana, F. excelsior*	bark	A	

Common Name	Botanical Name	Part Used	Safety Rating	Notes
white mulberry	*Morus alba*	root bark, twig, leaf, fruit	A	galactogogue
white pine	*Pinus strobus*	bark	A	
white sage	*Artemisia ludoviciana*	leaf	C	antigalactogogue; allergenic; toxicity potential unknown
wild cherry	*Prunus serotina*	bark	C	
wild ginger	*Asarum canadense*	rhizome	E	
wild hydrangea	*Hydrangea arborescens*	root, leaf	C	
wild indigo	*Baptisia tinctoria*	root, leaf	B	
wild lettuce	*Lactuca quercina, L. serriola, L. virosa*	leaf, stem	A	galactogogue; allergenic (rare)
wild oat	*Avena fatua*	seed head	A	
wild yam	*Dioscorea villosa*	rhizome	B	galactogogue; endangered
willow	*Salix alba*	bark	B	allergenic
winter savory	*Satureja montana*	leaf	A	
wintergreen	*Gaultheria procumbens*	fruit, essential oil	C	allergenic; essential oil is potentially toxic
wood betony	*Stachys officinalis*	leaf, stem	A	
wormseed (epazote)	*Chenopodium ambrosioides*	leaf, stem, seed oil	C, herb; E, seed oil	galactogogue; seed oil is toxic; contact allergenic

Common Name	Botanical Name	Part Used	Safety Rating	Notes
wormwood	*Artemisia absinthium*	leaf, stem	E	galactogogue?; essential oil is toxic
wu wei zi	*Schisandra chinensis*	fruit	A	
yarrow	*Achillea millefolium*	leaf, stem	B	antigalactogogue?; allergenic
yellow dock	*Rumex crispus, R. obtusifolius*	root	B	
yellow jessamine	*Gelsemium sempervirens*	root	E	
yerba maté	*Ilex paraguayensis*	leaf	B	stimulant (caffeine)
yerba santa	*Eriodictyon californicum, E. tomentosum*	leaf, stem	A	
yu zhu	*Polygonatum odoratum*	rhizome	A	
yucca	*Yucca aloifolia, Y. brevifolia, Y. glauca, Y. whipplei*	root	A	
zhi mu	*Anemarrhena asphodeloides*	rhizome	A	
zhi zi	*Gardenia jasminoides*	fruit	A	
zhu ling	*Grifola umbellata*	fruiting body, mycelium	A	

Galactogogue Herb Profiles

The following profiles offer thumbnail sketches of the most widely used galactogogue herbs. Each description lists the herb's common name, followed by its botanical name (in italics) and family name (in parentheses). While these herbs may have many uses unrelated to breastfeeding, they are commonly used by lactation consultants and lactation-specialist pediatricians in clinical practice. They have a tradition of galactogogue use among herbalists as well.

Many mothers find these herbs to be safe and effective with few side effects, most of which involve allergic reactions or diarrhea in the mother. I have noted known safety considerations for each herb, particularly as identified by the German Commission E and the American Herbal Products Association (AHPA). Both organizations use a panel of experts to evaluate herbs. Their findings reflect clinical experience as well as a consistent and extensive review of the scientific literature.

Note the allergic risk presented in each profile. If you or the baby's father have allergies or other hypersensitivity conditions, you should avoid herbs that are potentially allergenic. Or, take only a small amount of an herb, then wait twenty-four hours before consuming large amounts or combining it with other herbs. If you have an allergic reaction after drinking tea made with a combination of herbs, it may be hard to trace the reaction back to the culprit.

I have included directions for making tea from most of the herbs listed. (For larger quantities and galactogogue recipes, please see chapter 7.) The doses listed reflect either traditional usage or current recommendations for increasing milk supply. These doses have been drawn from a number of sources, not all of which agree. Although most of these herbs are widely available, health-food stores are the best place to look for bulk herbs and specialty products. In appendix B, you'll find contact information for companies that sell hard-to-find herbs, tinctures, and teas made specifically for increasing milk.

Herbs alone will not magically fix your breastfeeding problems. Before assuming that you do not have enough milk, consult with a lactation specialist. A fussy baby who appears hungry may, in fact, be reacting to oversupply, a forceful let-down, or other problems that could be made worse with galactogogue herbs. A lactation specialist can help you determine if you truly have a low milk supply and suggest ways to remedy your situation. If you know you need to increase your milk supply, there are basic remedial steps you must take: improving your baby's latch, for example, or starting to express milk. Many mothers find that these actions are sufficient and herbs are not needed. Remember, herbs can only aid lactation; they are not a cure-all. In some situations they can help mothers achieve or maintain a higher milk supply than would otherwise be possible. They have helped to bring in milk for adoptive mothers, women who have had breast reduction surgery, and those who have had a slow start breastfeeding and a persistently low supply. Whatever your situation, keep in touch with your lactation specialist as you work to build your milk.

You should also keep your baby's doctor informed of any herb usage, especially if you are using a formula supplement or if your baby has inadequate weight gain. If you are unable to nurse your baby or express enough milk, it may be essential to supplement your milk with formula. As more of your milk becomes available, you can reduce the formula with the help of your lactation consultant. Keep your doctor informed of your progress. If you or your baby has a health condition, or if you are using medications, consult your doctor and a knowledgeable herbalist before using any herb. For more about herbs and milk supply, see chapter 7.

alfalfa—*Medicago sativa* L. (Fabaceae)

> *Part used*: Aerial parts (stem, leaf, flower).
>
> *Tradition*: Argentinean, European herbalism.
>
> *Taste*: Bland, pleasant vegetable. Alfalfa leaf is an agreeable addition to tea blends.
>
> *Safety*: The German Commission E has not reviewed alfalfa. The AHPA labels alfalfa Class 1: safe when used appropriately. Experts have noted that alfalfa seeds contain canavanine, an alkaloid that has induced systemic lupus erythematosus (SLE) in laboratory animals. Although neither the plant nor the sprouts contains canavanine, SLE patients may prefer to avoid alfalfa entirely. In the dose range used for lactation, alfalfa may cause diarrhea. If it does, reduce the dose. Herbalist Mechell Turner recommends that women who take alfalfa during pregnancy discontinue use for the first five days after birth to reduce the chance of oversupply of milk.
>
> *Allergy*: Allergic reactions to alfalfa are not known. Alfalfa is a member of the pea family (Fabaceae), which includes many allergenic plants.
>
> *Dose*: Turner suggests starting with 1 tablet of alfalfa 4 times daily, working up to 8 tablets per day. If loose stools develop in mother or baby,

reduce the dose. To make a cup of tea, use 1–2 tablespoons (3.8–7.5 g) dried leaves per 5 oz. (150 mL) boiling water. Drink up to 1 quart a day. To make a quart, combine 1–2 oz. (30–60 g) with 1 quart of boiling water; steep overnight. Or take 1 tablespoon dried juice powder 2 times per day. Alfalfa is used in large amounts in combination recipes.
Availability: Dried alfalfa is available in bulk and in simple capsules. Expressed juice is available at health-food stores in various forms (look in the "green foods" or "liquid chlorophyll" section). Extracts can be purchased in capsules or pressed tablets. Sprouts are widely available.

anise—*Pimpinella anisum* L. (Apiaceae)
Part used: Seed (botanically a fruit).
Tradition: European herbalism. In the Netherlands, cookies with anise seed are a traditional gift to new mothers to ensure bountiful milk.
Taste: Sweet.
Safety: The German Commission E has approved use of the seed for indigestion and coughs. There are no known contraindications or interactions with other medicines. Some people are allergic to anethole, the aromatic part of anise. The AHPA lists anise as Class 2b: not to be used during pregnancy. Anise has been used as an emmenagogue. Note that star anise and anise are entirely different plants. Star anise is not a safe substitute for anise; herbal products containing star anise may be contaminated by the toxic Japanese star anise, which looks similar to star anise. Japanese star anise is often used in potpourri.
Allergy: The anethole found in anise seed has caused occasional allergic reactions of the skin, gastrointestinal tract, and respiratory tract.
Dose: To make tea, cover 1–2 teaspoons (3.5–7 g) freshly crushed seed with 5 oz. (150 mL) boiling water. Steep, tightly covered, for 10–20 minutes. Take up to 5–6 times a day. Anise is often combined with other herbs, particularly other aromatic seeds.
Availability: Whole seeds are available in grocery stores.

blessed thistle—*Cnicus benedictus* L. (Asteraceae)
Part used: Blooming plant (stem, leaf, and flower).
Tradition: European herbalism.
Taste: Bitter.

Safety: The German Commission E has approved blessed thistle for indigestion and loss of appetite. The plant stimulates the secretion of saliva and gastric juices when used in a dose of 4–6 g/day. There are no known interactions with other drugs. Individuals who are allergic to plants in the Asteraceae family should avoid blessed thistle. Do not use blessed thistle during pregnancy. The AHPA labels blessed thistle Class 1: safe when used appropriately. No side effects have been identified in nursing infants, though maternal diarrhea has occurred (rare). Therefore, a similar reaction in infants is possible.

Allergy: As a member of the Asteraceae family, blessed thistle is a potential allergen. The German Commission E notes that no allergic reactions have been reported.

Dose: Take 3 capsules dried herb (250–300 mg each) 3 times per day (up to 2–3 g/day) when combined with fenugreek, or take up to 6 g/day in divided doses when used alone. To make tea, cover 1–2 teaspoons (1–2 g) dried herb with 5 oz. (150 mL) boiling water and steep for 5–10 minutes. Or place the dried herb in cold water, bring to a boil, and immediately remove from heat. Sweeten as needed, but keep in mind that the bitter taste will best stimulate your digestive juices. Drink up to 5–6 times per day. Moderate amounts of blessed thistle are used in recipes.

Availability: Available at health-food stores in bulk, capsules, or combination teas.

caraway—*Carum carvi* L. (Apiaceae)

Part used: Seed (botanically a fruit), essential oil.

Tradition: European herbalism.

Taste: More savory than sweet; pleasant and aromatic.

Safety: The German Commission E has approved the use of caraway seed (1.5–6 g/day) and essential oil (3–6 drops/day) for bloating, fullness, and mild spasms of the gastrointestinal tract. Caraway has also been used to treat colic in infants. There are no known contraindications, adverse effects, or drug interactions. The AHPA had labeled caraway Class 1: safe when used appropriately.

Allergy: Unlike the allergenic members of the Apiaceae family, caraway essential oil does not contain the allergen anethole. The aromatic component is mostly carvone, which is considered nonallergenic. No allergic reactions have been reported.

Dose: To make tea, combine 1–2 teaspoons (3.5–7 g) freshly crushed seeds in 5 oz. (150 mL) boiling water; cover tightly and steep for 10–20 minutes. Strain. Drink warm up to 5–6 times a day. Caraway is often combined with other herbs, particularly other aromatic seeds.

Availability: Widely available in grocery stores. Caraway is part of a traditional German galactogogue tea product, which is now available in the United States. (See appendix B.)

chasteberry—*Vitex agnus-castus* L. (Verbenaceae)

Part used: Fruit, leaf.

Tradition: European herbalism. The fruit has been used since antiquity to increase milk. In Roman times, the leaf was used to speed delivery of the child and placenta, and to "bring down" the milk. Throughout history, the fruit has been used in maintaining the chastity of monks and as an all-purpose women's herb throughout the Mediterranean region.

Taste: Peppery.

Safety: The German Commission E has approved chasteberry for irregularities of the menstrual cycle and for premenstrual complaints, including breast pain. The editors state that there are no toxicity issues. Chasteberry is thought to have a dopaminergic effect on the pituitary. It is widely used in England and Germany for most menstrual irregularities and PMS symptoms. The fruit improves corpus luteum activity, establishing normal levels of progesterone in the menstrual cycle and normalizing the frequency of the menstrual period. Although chasteberry is not known to have adverse effects on breastfeeding infants, recent literature cautions against using chasteberry while breastfeeding. In animal studies, chasteberry lowers prolactin response, and, when administered in large injected doses, it suppresses lactation in rats. Short-term studies of men have shown that small doses (120 mg/day) of chasteberry increase prolactin release while large doses (500 mg/day) lower prolactin release. Dose-response studies for women are lacking. Chasteberry was the first galactogogue herb to be investigated with breastfeeding women. Although preliminary studies, conducted in Germany during the 1940s and 1950s, showed a positive effect, no modern studies have been done. There is insufficient data to say whether chasteberry should be used to increase milk, yet such traditional use continues. It may be that the short-term effect of chasteberry is to increase prolactin and milk flow; however, using even small doses of chasteberry continuously for several weeks may reverse lactation amenorrhea, which is an important benefit of breastfeeding. Chasteberry is known to promote fertility. In clinical trials, previously infertile women have become pregnant after several months' therapy with chasteberry. Some breastfeeding women use chasteberry to hasten the return of menses in order to achieve fertility without weaning. The AHPA lists chasteberry as Class 2b: seek expert help before use during pregnancy. (Seek expert medical and herbalist guidance before discontinuing chasteberry if you have become pregnant through its use, however.) The fruit can cause gastrointestinal upset, headache, or allergic rash (rare). Chasteberry should not be used with synthetic fertility drugs; it could also possibly interfere with drugs that block dopamine (including domperidone, metoclopramide, haloperidol).

Allergy: Itching and rash (rare).

Dose: In Germany, doses used for PMS and irregular menses are typically low (the equivalent of 30–40 mg per day of the fruit, usually in tincture or solid extract forms). Most studies have shown efficacy in treating menstrual disturbances with these low doses, which were the approximate doses used in the original breastfeeding studies. In English-speaking countries, higher doses (ranging from a 175 mg capsule taken once a day to 500 mg capsules taken twice a day) are often used for menstrual disturbances. To increase milk supply, try alternative herbs first. Use chasteberry in small doses (30–40 mg/day) and for short periods of time, especially in the early weeks of lactation.

Availability: Many dried extract and tincture products are available in Germany, where the herb is a top seller. Tinctures are widely available in the United States and may be easier to use in small doses, which are safest for lactation. One company provides a standardized product from Germany in a larger dose (175 mg capsules), which is suitable for regulating periods and regaining fertility. (See appendix B.)

dill—*Anethum graveolens* L. (Apiaceae)

Part used: Seed, essential oil.

Tradition: Indian, European, and Middle Eastern herbalism.

Taste: Sweet with savory overtones.

Safety: The German Commission E has approved essential oil and dill seed for indigestion; it notes no contraindications or restrictions. Dill is a component of gripewater, which is used to treat colic in infants. The AHPA rates the seed Class 1: safe when used appropriately.

Allergy: Although dill is a member of the allergenic Apiaceae family, the seed oil does not contain the allergen anethole. The aromatic component is mostly carvone, which is considered nonallergenic.

Dose: To make tea, combine 1 teaspoon (2.5 g) freshly crushed seed per 5 oz. (150 mL) boiling water. Cover tightly and steep 10–20 minutes. Strain and drink warm up to 5–6 times a day. Dill is often combined with other herbs, especially other aromatic seeds.

Availability: Dill seed is available in grocery stores.

fennel—*Foeniculum vulgare* Mill. (Apiaceae)

Part used: Seed (botanically a fruit), essential oil.

Tradition: European herbalism.

Taste: Sweet.

Safety: The German Commission E has found fennel seed effective for mild indigestion and coughs in doses up to 5–7 g/day. It notes no restriction for use of the seed, but states that the essential oil should not be used during pregnancy or with infants or small children. The AHPA considers fennel Class 1: safe when used appropriately. It notes that fennel essential oil contains significant levels of the toxin estragole. The editors state that, in appropriate doses, this estragole is immediately metabolized in the liver, meaning it does not enter general blood circulation and therefore will not reach the breast. They go on to state that only prolonged use or excessive doses of fennel would allow the estragole to get past the liver and into the bloodstream. So, in appropriate doses, estragole is not expected to enter the breast milk; the baby would be exposed to estragole only if directly fed fennel products. The AHPA notes no known drug interactions for fennel. Note: Fennel has several toxic, look-alike relatives, including water parsnip, cow parsnip, and hemlock. Socrates was executed with a drink of hemlock *(Conium maculatum)*, which looks a lot like fennel. Know your source. Every so often, someone is poisoned after ingesting one of fennel's cousins, picked in the wild. Do not use fennel continuously for more than a few weeks without consulting your doctor. Do not exceed the recommended dose, especially of the essential oil. Excessive doses of fennel may have contributed to adverse reactions in two newborn babies. The mothers had consumed 2 quarts per day of tea (twice the appropriate dose), reportedly with fennel and other herbs; however, the actual plants were never formally identified. It is possible that a toxic relative of fennel had been consumed in large amounts.

Allergy: Fennel contains anethole, which occasionally causes allergic reactions of the skin, gastrointestinal tract, and respiratory tract.

Dose: To make tea, combine 1–3 teaspoons (2.5–7.5 g) freshly crushed seeds and 8 oz. (250 mL) boiling water. Cover tightly and steep 10–20 minutes. Take up to 5–6 times per day. To make a strong standard infusion, combine 4–8 tablespoons (30–60 g) fennel seed per quart of boiling water. Take up to 3–4 cups a day. Fennel is best when freshly crushed. It is usually used in lower doses when combined with other herbs. Fennel is often combined with other aromatic seeds.

Availability: Whole seed is available in grocery stores.

fenugreek—*Trigonella foenum-graecum* L. (Fabaceae)

Part used: Seed. (In India, the leaf and seed oil are also used to increase milk.)

Tradition: Ayurvedic origin, spreading to the Middle East and Europe.

Taste: Bitter taste, with a smell somewhere between strong celery seed and maple syrup.

Safety: The German Commission E has approved fenugreek for internal use as an appetite stimulant. It reports that no contraindications or drug interactions are known. The Commission notes that external use may cause an allergic skin reaction. The AHPA labels fenugreek Class 2b: seek expert help before use during pregnancy. It notes no other warnings. High doses of fenugreek may lower blood sugar slightly (15–100 g/day ingested whole seed is used as complementary treatment for diabetes), but galactogogue dose ranges are often much smaller (3–5 g/day) and hypoglycemic symptoms in the mother are not anticipated. However, some stimulation of appetite may be expected when consuming whole seeds in the higher dose ranges used for teas (1–2 oz., or

30–60 g, per day). The sudden introduction of fenugreek into the diet will sometimes cause diarrhea in the mother and (even more rarely) in the baby. Reducing the dose or slowing introduction into the diet reverses this diarrhea.

Allergy: Repeated inhalation of the powdered seed has induced asthma in factory workers. Using fenugreek may exacerbate existing asthma; mothers with asthma or allergic tendencies should avoid the powdered forms, including capsules. Cases of contact dermatitis have been noted even with first-time external use, so avoid fenugreek if you are allergic to peanuts, soy, or other members of the pea family (Fabaceae).

Dose: Fenugreek is the most widely used galactogogue in the West; numerous dosages and preparations are used. Ayurvedic and Egyptian references describe a dose of 3–6 g per day fenugreek seeds, often made into porridge with cow's milk, pressed into cakes with honey (soak the seeds first), or ground and steeped as a tea or decoction. The usual North American recommendation is up to 3 g/day fenugreek in divided doses (for example, a 1 g capsule 3 times a day). This may not be a sufficient dose for some women. Start with 1 g/day in divided doses and increase the dose until your sweat and milk smell like maple syrup. Dr. Jack Newman considers this a reliable method for achieving an effective dose. To make tea, steep 1–3 teaspoons (4.5–13.5 g) whole seed in 8 oz. (250 mL) boiling water for 5–10 minutes or longer, then sweeten. Drink 2–4 times a day. (Whole seeds require higher doses than crushed seeds. If you wish to grind the seeds first, reduce the total amount of seed used. Note that ground seeds will make the tea—and the taste—stronger.) Alternatively, whole seeds can be soaked in cold water for 3 hours, then strained. The tea should be heated gently before drinking. Women have also reported success after eating whole seeds soaked overnight in a small amount of water. You might also make a decoction with the whole seeds, then add other herbs such as fennel or anise to improve the taste and effect. Some lactation consultants find fenugreek tincture to be more consistently effective than other preparations. Recommended tincture doses vary according to the product, so follow the label instructions carefully. Herbalist Mechell Turner suggests 3 mL 3 times daily. Herbalist Tammy Karnes suggests taking 30 drops every 2–3 hours for 48 hours, then reducing this to 30 drops 4 times daily. Herbalist

Kathryn Higgins suggests 3–4 drops for every 10 lbs. of the mother's body weight, taken every other hour (except when sleeping); this can be reduced to 3–4 times a day after milk supply increases, which generally occurs after 1–2 days.

Availability: Capsules of ground seed are widely available. Fenugreek capsule sizes vary from 250 to 1200 mg, so you must figure out how many capsules to take based on the doses listed here. Avoid defatted or debittered forms, as it is not known which constituents are important for increasing milk. The oil and bitter constituents probably contribute to galactogogue activity. Avoid thyme-fenugreek combination capsules, as these are designed for other uses and offer an insufficient dose of fenugreek. Fenugreek galactogogue tinctures are available in single and combination forms. (See appendix B.)

goat's rue—*Galega officinalis* L. (Fabaceae)

Part used: Dried blooming plant (stem, leaf, flower).

Tradition: European herbalism, animal husbandry. (In France, the plant is fed to dairy animals to increase milk yield.)

Taste: May be disagreeably bitter.

Safety: Goat's rue is used in folk medicine to lower blood sugar, but because evidence of efficacy is lacking, the German Commission E has not approved goat's rue for the treatment of diabetes. Poisoning has occurred in animals grazing on the fresh plant; however, dried goat's rue has long been fed to dairy animals to increase milk production. Some consider the fresh plant to be toxic. A combination product containing goat's rue is reported to have caused an adverse reaction in nursing infants, but the report is very incomplete. The AHPA has not reviewed goat's rue.

Allergy: Although goat's rue is a member of the pea family (Fabaceae), no allergic reactions have been reported.

Dose: There is no consensus on dosage for this plant. For a cup of tea, *Herbal Drugs and Phytopharmaceuticals* (often referred to as the "Teedrogen") recommends a scant $1/2$–1 teaspoon (0.5–1 g) dried flower tops with 5 oz. (150 mL) boiling water; drink 3–5 times a day. For a decoction, boil 1 scant teaspoon per 5 oz. (150 mL) water for 2–3 minutes, then cool. Take 4–5 times a day. English herbalist David Hoffmann suggests fewer doses of stronger tea per day to increase milk: use 1 teaspoon (about 1 g) dried herb in 8 oz. (250 mL) water; steep for 10–15 minutes and take 2 times daily. In France, where goat's rue is most commonly used, some lactation specialists recommend large amounts (30–60 g per quart) to start. Steep for 10–15 minutes at most before straining. Single and combination tinctures are also available to increase milk supply; follow the directions printed on the label. Goat's rue is used in small to moderate amounts in recipes.

Availability: Fresh goat's rue is not generally grown in the United States and seeds are not available for sale due to the herb's noxious weed status. The dried herb and galactogogue tinctures are available through specialty herb companies. (See appendix B.)

hops—*Humulus lupulus* L. (Moraceae)

Part used: Strobilus (conelike flowering part).

Tradition: European herbalism. English tradition suggests that nursing mothers drink a bottle of dark beer or stout in the late afternoon to help build their milk supply and to relax. (Beer gets much of its bitter taste from hops.) Dried hops are used in sleep pillows (aromatherapy).

Taste: Strong, spicy, and bitter.

Safety: The German Commission E has approved a single dose of hops (0.5 g) per day for mood disturbances such as restlessness, anxiety, and sleeplessness. The Commission reports no contraindications or drug interactions. The AHPA labels hops as Class 2d, noting that some herbalists caution against using the herb during depression due to its mildly sedative properties. Otherwise the AHPA lists no contraindications or drug interactions.

Allergy: None reported.

Dose: Hops is considered by herbalists to be relatively "harsh" for breastfeeding mothers. However, in small doses, hops is considered helpful in triggering a reluctant let-down. It makes a bitter tea: For a single cup of tea, steep 1 scant teaspoon (about 0.5 g) dried herb in 5 oz. (150 mL) boiling water for 10–15 minutes; drink no more than 2 cups a day. Small quantities of hops are used in recipes.

Availability: Bulk quantities are sometimes available in natural food stores.

marshmallow—*Althaea officinalis* L. (Malvaceae)

Part used: Root.

Tradition: European herbalism. Marshmallow has also been used as food; it was once widely consumed as the original marshmallow candy.

Taste: Sweetish; the tea and low-alcoholic tinctures are mucilaginous.

Safety: The German Commission E has approved the internal use of marshmallow root powder to treat dry coughs as well as mouth, throat, and stomach irritations. There are no known contraindications. Marshmallow root may slow the absorption of other drugs due to its mucilaginous nature. The AHPA labels marshmallow root Class 1: safe when used appropriately.

Allergy: None reported.

Dose: To make tea, pour 5 oz. (150 mL) cold water over 1 tablespoon (15 g) root powder; let it stand for 30 minutes, stirring frequently. Strain and heat the tea gently before drinking. Drink several times per day. Marshmallow root tea is best when prepared fresh each time. Use it quickly, as the tea soon becomes too thick to drink easily, especially if powdered root is used. To prevent a gooey mess when mixing marshmallow in quart recipes, use root pieces or only small amounts of powdered root. To make a decoction, combine 4 tablespoons (60 g) root powder or 4 handfuls of root pieces with 1 quart of water; bring to a boil and simmer. Reduce the volume by 1/4, then strain and cool. The decoction will keep well when refrigerated. However you choose to take it, marshmallow is probably best when combined with other herbs. It can also counter the bowel-loosening effects of herbs such as alfalfa, fenugreek, or blessed thistle while adding a sweet taste. To use, add about 4 oz. of marshmallow decoction to each dose of a standard infusion tea, then warm gently. Marshmallow is also used externally to create a soothing and slippery massage bath to help trigger milk let-down or ease plugged ducts. Add enough marshmallow to make the hot water slippery.

Availability: Bulk quantities are sometimes available in natural food stores. Marshmallow root is used in commercial galactogogue teas. Powdered root is available in capsules, although it would take many capsules per day to match the amount used in tea.

milk thistle—*Silybum marianum* L. Gaertn. (Asteraceae)

Part used: Stem, seed. (Traditionally, the peeled, tender shoots have been used as food and to increase milk supply.)

Tradition: European herbalism.

Taste: Seeds are oily and bitter; they should not taste or smell rancid.

Safety: The German Commission E notes an occasional mild laxative effect with milk thistle. No other side effects, contraindications, or drug interactions have been identified. The AHPA considers milk thistle Class 1: safe when used appropriately.

Allergy: Although a member of the Asteraceae family, no allergic reactions have been reported.

Dose: To make tea, use 1 heaping teaspoon (3–5 g) freshly chopped seeds in 5 oz. (150 mL) boiling water; steep 20–30 minutes. Take up to 5–6 times a day. Standardized milk thistle products are widely available and are mainly used for liver conditions. As there is no specific information on galactogogue use, carefully follow doses printed on product labels. Although these products are concentrated, no adverse effects have been noted in nursing mothers or their infants.

Availability: Standardized seed extracts and powdered seed capsules are available in health-food stores. Fresh, whole seeds are preferable to powdered seed capsules.

raspberry—*Rubus idaeus* L. (Rosaceae)

Part used: Leaf.

Tradition: North American, European, Asian herbalism.

Taste: Slightly harsh and bitter with a hint of floral flavor.

Safety: Although the German Commission E could not identify any risks associated with raspberry leaf, it has not approved its use because no studies of efficacy could be found. Regardless, raspberry leaf is extensively used during pregnancy to prepare for labor and breastfeeding. For most women, it is unnecessary to use this or any other herb during pregnancy to make sufficient milk, but prenatal use does not seem to overstimulate supply or contribute to engorgement in the postpartum. Raspberry leaf contains tannins and is thought to be somewhat astringent. It is believed to lower milk supply with long-term use in the postpartum, even though it seems to increase supply when used short-term (less than a week). It is best to use raspberry leaf only briefly and as a minor part of galactogogue recipes. The AHPA labels raspberry leaf Class 1: safe when used appropriately. It notes no restrictions.

Allergy: None reported.

Dose: To make tea, combine 1 teaspoon (0.8 g) finely chopped dried leaf per 5 oz. (150 mL) boiling water; steep for 5 minutes. The tea may become bitter with a longer steeping time. Some women consume 1 quart of tea per day during pregnancy; smaller amounts should be used during breastfeeding. Use raspberry for no more than a week when trying to build your milk supply. Small amounts of raspberry leaf are used in combination with other herbs in recipes. Raspberry leaf is also used in commercial tea products. (See appendix B.)

Availability: Teas and bulk quantities are generally available in natural food stores.

stinging nettle—*Urtica dioica* L., *U. urens* L. (Urticaceae)

Part used: Blooming plant (leaf, stem, flower).

Tradition: European herbalism.

Taste: Pleasant vegetable taste in tea; tasty vegetable once cooked. The dried or cooked plant does not sting.

Safety: The German Commission E has approved use of the leaf as supportive therapy for rheumatic ailments, urinary tract infections, and for preventing and treating small kidneys stones. The Commission lists no contraindications, drug interactions, or side effects for the leaf. The AHPA considers stinging nettle Class 1: safe when used appropriately. Wear gloves when handling fresh young plants.

Allergy: Rare cases of allergic dermatitis or stomach irritation have been reported in patients after taking nettle tea.

Dose: Freshly picked stinging nettle can be eaten as a steamed vegetable. To make tea, combine 3–4 teaspoons (4 g) dried herb with 5 oz. (150 mL) boiling water; steep 10 minutes. (Or place in cold water, boil for 5 minutes, and remove from heat.) Take up to 5–6 times a day. Nettle tea is often made a quart at a time (use up to 60 g per quart; infuse overnight), and large amounts are often combined with other herbs. Capsules of powdered or freeze-dried leaf are widely available (freeze-dried nettle relieves symptoms of hay fever). To increase milk supply, many capsules would be needed to achieve a sufficient dose. Nettle tincture is notably effective in simple or combination forms.

Availability: Health-food stores are the best place to find a range of nettle products: bulk dried stinging nettle, capsules of dried or freeze-dried nettle, and specialty tinctures. See appendix B for nettle tinctures and teas specifically developed for lactation.

vervain—*Verbena officinalis* L. (Verbenaceae)

Part used: Blooming plant (leaf, stem, flower).

Tradition: First Nations in North America, European herbalism.

Taste: Bitter and sharp.

Safety: Due to insufficient data on efficacy, the German Commission E has not approved vervain for medicinal use. The editors state that there are no known toxicity issues. The United States has classified vervain as an Herb of Undefined Safety. The plant contains verbenalin, which, in extremely high doses, can cause stupor and seizures in animals. These toxic effects have not been seen in humans using the whole herb. The PDR *(Physician's Desk Reference)* for herbal medicine lists no health hazards or side effects when vervain is used appropriately. (The PDR gives no dose range.) The AHPA labels vervain as Class 2b: seek expert help before use during pregnancy. Vervain has shown galactogogue and oxytocic activity, and it is found to be uterotonic in animals.

Allergy: No allergic reactions reported.

Dose: To make tea, steep 1 teaspoon (1.5 g) dried herb in 5 oz. (150 mL) boiling water for 5–10 minutes. Take up to 5–6 times a day. In Europe, a stronger infusion is used to stimulate milk supply: combine a handful (6–10 tablespoons, or 30–50 g) of vervain with a quart of boiling water. Steep for 10–15 minutes. Reduce this dose as milk increases. Vervain is used in moderate amounts in recipes.

Availability: Not widely available as a single product in stores; look for bulk products. Vervain is usually combined with other herbs in galactogogue teas or tinctures. (See appendix B.)

*I*ndex